Free DVD 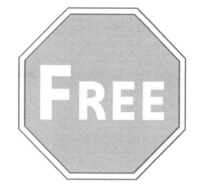 **Free DVD**

Essential Test Tips DVD from Trivium Test Prep

Dear Customer,

Thank you for purchasing from Trivium Test Prep! Whether you're looking to join the military, get into college, or advance your career, we're honored to be a part of your journey.

To show our appreciation (and to help you relieve a little of that test-prep stress), we're offering a **FREE *ACSM Essential Test Tips DVD*** by Trivium Test Prep. Our DVD includes 35 test preparation strategies that will help keep you calm and collected before and during your big exam. All we ask is that you email us your feedback and describe your experience with our product. Amazing, awful, or just so-so: we want to hear what you have to say!

To receive your **FREE *ACSM Essential Test Tips DVD***, please email us at 5star@ triviumtestprep.com. Include "Free 5 Star" in the subject line and the following information in your email:

1. The title of the product you purchased.

2. Your rating from 1 – 5 (with 5 being the best).

3. Your feedback about the product, including how our materials helped you meet your goals and ways in which we can improve our products.

4. Your full name and shipping address so we can send your **FREE *ACSM Essential Test Tips DVD***.

If you have any questions or concerns please feel free to contact us directly at 5star@triviumtestprep.com.

Thank you, and good luck with your studies!

ACSM CERTIFICATION PRACTICE TESTS

Personal Training Exam Review Book with Over 400 Practice Test Questions for the Academy of Sports Medicine CPT Test

About the Authors

Beth Lazarou just celebrated her sixth year as a National Academy of Sports Medicine (NASM)-certified personal trainer. She is also a certified Group Fitness Instructor through the American Council on Exercise (ACE), a NASM Fitness Nutrition Specialist, and a NASM Corrective Exercise Specialist. In addition, Beth holds a Kettlebell Instruction Certification through the American Sports and Fitness Association. She specializes in social, HIIT, kettlebell, and functional fitness. Currently, Beth is attending Arizona State University's online program, pursuing a BS in Health Science.

Keith Lee Schuchardt received a BS in Exercise Science: Fitness Specialist from West Chester University of Pennsylvania. He went on to obtain an MS in Exercise Science: Health Promotion and Rehabilitation Science from California University of Pennsylvania. Keith has been certified through the National Strength and Conditioning Association (NSCA) as a Certified Strength and Conditioning Specialist, the National Academy of Sports Medicine (NASM) as a Corrective Exercise Specialist, and the American College of Sports Medicine (ACSM) as a Certified Exercise Physiologist. For over a decade, he has worked as a personal trainer in both corporate and private settings, as well as a strength and conditioning coach for professional and collegiate athletes. He is currently pursuing a Doctorate in Physical Therapy at A.T. Still University.

TABLE OF CONTENTS

INTRODUCTION

What is a Personal Trainer?

The world of personal training is vast and growing in many ways. A personal trainer is an educated exercise professional who possesses the knowledge and skill set to create and instruct others in various fitness-related settings. Personal trainers must strive to achieve a base of knowledge and to acquire the skills to properly design and implement research-based training programs that are safe and effective for their clientele. It is up to the certified personal trainer to ensure the client receives the highest quality training experience through appropriate goal setting, needs analysis, exercise prescriptions, and health and fitness education. Additionally, it is the certified personal trainer's responsibility to develop and employ these methods within his or her scope of practice. There are a variety of different career paths a certified personal trainer can pursue based on his or her interests and abilities.

Personal trainers can be productive in many different settings and businesses. The most common settings in which personal trainers work are the large, well-known gym chains and smaller, privately owned fitness centers that are common in the United States. These facilities are generally open to hiring newly trained, certified fitness professionals and are a good starting point for anyone looking to advance within a specific company.

However, there are a number of other settings in which certified personal trainers can utilize their health and fitness knowledge. For example, personal trainers can work in clinical settings, corporate training, in-home private settings, sports camps, and more. Working in a clinical setting as a personal trainer often involves administering exercise stress tests with a team supervised by a physician or medical practitioner. Corporate trainers tend to work at the private fitness centers of corporations in an office building. Some clientele prefer a more personalized workout within the privacy of their own home; the certified personal trainer will travel to the client's house with his or her equipment. Depending on the fitness professional's background, it may be preferable to work as a sports-specific strength and conditioning coach. There are many career paths available, but one key component of the personal training world is the certification.

Getting Certified

BENEFITS OF CERTIFICATION

Earning a certification through a nationally recognized fitness organization is one of the most important accomplishments for a fitness professional aiming to further his or her career. Certification is important for several reasons. First, fitness certifications require the acquisition of a substantial amount of valuable expertise and knowledge to pass the examination. Second, maintenance of most certifications requires continuing education through conventions, seminars, or other educational opportunities, so professionals keep their knowledge current and stay abreast of trends in the field. Finally, certification through major organizations demonstrates credibility to peers and clientele. The examination process requires adequate preparation to ensure successful candidates become personal trainers.

Fitness certification exams test individuals on a wide variety of exercise-science-based concepts. The concepts tested include, but are not limited to: exercise physiology, biomechanics, exercise psychology, anatomy and physiology, exercise prescription and program design, fitness facility organization and management, fitness programs for various populations, and more. Various fitness organizations provide test preparation materials such as study guides, review books, and practice tests that provide individuals with an idea of what they should expect on the exam. Fitness professionals seeking to become certified must prepare themselves for the exam by studying and being able to apply the knowledge in the materials. The certification exams are intentionally difficult in order to adequately prepare the candidates to work as competent professionals in the field of exercise science. This ensures the certified personal trainer will provide clients with safe and effective fitness programs.

Maintaining a fitness certification through the major organizations requires continued educational pursuits among the various topics in exercise science. This can be achieved through many avenues such as fitness conventions, web seminars, informational sessions with accompanying tests, and additional certifications. The purpose of continuing education credits for certifications is to ensure that the certified personal trainer maintains current knowledge and relevant expertise. Ever-improving scientific testing protocols, procedures, and equipment optimize the data that fitness professionals use to create ideal programs for clients. Studying the most up-to-date material ensures that the client is provided the most efficient method for obtaining their goals, but it is up to the trainer to guide them in the correct direction.

Credibility among trainers is ensured through the aforementioned certification process. Clientele and employers who are seeking the most qualified candidate can be assured they have a professional trainer by the certification the trainer holds. Based on the strenuous testing protocol and ongoing education requirements, certification makes it easier to determine whether a trainer is ready for a gig. High-profile employers will often require elite certifications of their training staff. For instance, professional sports teams often insist on a specific certification before considering an applicant. This requirement is often common at the collegiate level of fitness professionals as well. It shows the employers that the trainer has taken the time to understand the information relevant to providing the most effective program for their athletes.

It is highly important for individuals seeking any employment in the fitness industry to acquire certification through the major exercise organizations. The rigorous testing protocols require fitness professionals to achieve significant expertise in a variety of topics, which enhances their ability to create effective exercise programs. The major fitness organizations ensure fitness professionals keep their knowledge and expertise current. Certification supplies the employer and clients with an understanding of a fitness professional's level of credibility and competency in the field. In preparation for this great achievement, the fitness professional must first select which certification best fits his or her goals.

The following list provides information on some of the advantages and disadvantages for various major fitness certifications:

AMERICAN COUNCIL ON EXERCISE (ACE) CERTIFICATION

Advantages: The ACE certifications undergo accreditation through the National Commission for Certifying Agencies (NCCA), which ensures a program's certifications are evaluated for high-quality outcomes for their professionals. There are a variety of different certification specializations that can be obtained, which provides fitness professionals with different fields of expertise to study. ACE has an agreement for guaranteed interviews with several major fitness clubs that are found throughout the United States, enhancing the ability to find potential jobs. ACE certifications do not require a college-level degree to sit for the exam. All research utilized to develop the study material is scientifically evidence-based to ensure its effectiveness.

Disadvantages: The study materials and test can be expensive, totaling over $600 for the Personal Trainers Certification alone without specializations. Higher-profile training jobs, such as professional and collegiate strength coaches, typically require certification through other organizations such as ACSM or NSCA.

National Academy of Sports Medicine (NASM) Certification

Advantages: The NASM certifications are also accredited through the NCCA like ACE, ensuring credibility. NASM certifications also do not require a bachelor's degree to sit for examination. NASM offers a money-back guarantee in finding employment in the field within ninety days. The certification exams are difficult, but the material effectively prepares candidates for the test if studied adequately. There are a variety of different specializations to choose from, including corrective exercise, sports performance, youth training, and more. Many colleges and universities have partnered with NASM to supply certifications through classes offered at the schools.

Disadvantages: The study materials and exams are also expensive, ranging from $699 to $1,299 depending on what program is selected. The certifications do not require continuing education to maintain certification, which could potentially cause information to become obsolete.

National Strength and Conditioning Association (NSCA)—Certified Strength and Conditioning Specialist (CSCS)

Advantages: The NSCA is accredited through the NCCA like the previous two certifying organizations. The NSCA—Certified Strength and Conditioning Specialist exam is very well known nationally and with professional athletic organizations as one of the top fitness certifications. The CSCS certification is specifically designed for preparing exercise programs for athletes and improving sports performance. Another advantage is that there are numerous study sources for the exam, including a textbook, practice exams, online and classroom clinics, and test prep materials. Also, becoming a member of the organization reduces the cost of the exam itself, and the exam is slightly cheaper than the aforementioned certifications. The textbook is thorough and excellent preparation for the exam.

Disadvantages: The NSCA—CSCS certification exam is difficult and contains a large amount of information and requires a lot of preparation time. Furthermore, this specific certification requires that candidates either be currently enrolled as a senior or hold a bachelor's degree in exercise science. Finally, the study materials can become pricey if more than a textbook is required.

AMERICAN COLLEGE OF SPORTS MEDICINE (ACSM) CERTIFICATION

Advantages: Like the aforementioned certifications, the ACSM certifications are accredited through the NCCA. Also, like the NSCA, the ACSM is a highly recognized certifying fitness organization. There are multiple certifications available for those with backgrounds in exercise science (e.g., ACSM—Certified Exercise Physiologist) and those without (e.g., ACSM—Certified Personal Trainer). These certifications are designed to adequately prepare the fitness professional for exercise program design for general and special populations. The certification is excellent at teaching how to manage and stratify risks with new clientele. There are various modes of test preparation supplies similar to that of the NSCA.

Disadvantages: Some ACSM exams require a bachelor's degree in exercise science or a related field. They have a high degree of difficulty and the preparation materials and services can be expensive. Furthermore, employers may prefer other certifications depending on the type of clientele they work with. For example, although the ACSM is considered as a gold standard in fitness, professional athletic teams may seek NSCA—CSCS certified trainers because they specialize in sports performance.

It is in the best interest of the fitness professional to do as much research on the various certifications as possible. This includes researching the type of environment in which the fitness professional wants to advance their career. Selecting the right certification for a specified career path in fitness can help to save a lot of money and time in the long run. It may be necessary to look into specific employers to determine which type of training certification will improve the chances for success. Additionally, researching the testing procedures and requirements will help educate the fitness professional on the level of commitment required to become a certified trainer.

American College of Sports Medicine (ACSM): Introduction

The **American College of Sports Medicine (ACSM)** is another of the oldest professional fitness organizations in the field of exercise science and is recognized as a gold standard in health and fitness. Developed in the 1950s, the ACSM is a worldwide association of over 50,000 members. The organization was developed by physicians and fitness professionals working together to provide the highest-quality research in the field of sports medicine and exercise. The ACSM offers a variety of certifications for all levels of education and various specializations and credential programs. ACSM certifications include certified personal trainer (CPT), certified group exercise instructor (GEI), and certified exercise physiologist

(EP-C). ACSM advanced certifications include certified clinical exercise physiologist (CEP) requiring a bachelor's degree in exercise science and clinical work experience, as well as registered certified exercise physiologist (RCEP) requiring a graduate degree and experience overseeing clinical exercise testing. Like the NSCA, the ACSM has been devoted to producing science-based research journals in sports medicine and exercise science for decades and is seen as one of the leaders in fitness education worldwide. The main goal of the ACSM is to develop the most scientifically relevant research, methods, and application of their research to the entirety of the health and fitness industry.

ACSM Test Details

The ACSM tests are broken up into different domains testing various exercise-science–related aspects. The Certified Personal Trainer (ACSM—CPT) exam has 150 questions split into four testing domains: Initial Client Consultation and Assessment; Exercise Program Design and Implementation; Exercise Leadership and Client Education; and Legal, Professional, Business, and Marketing. Candidates have two hours and thirty minutes to complete the ACSM—CPT exam and receive test results immediately.

What's on the ACSM Certification Exams?		
Domain	Number of Questions	Percentage of Exam
Initial Client Consultation and Assessment	39	26%
Exercise Program Design and Implementation	41 (approx.)	27%
Exercise Leadership and Client Education	40 (approx.)	27%
Legal, Professional, Business, and Marketing	30	20%
Total:	150 questions	2 hours and 30 minutes

Questions in Domain I, Initial Client Consultation and Assessment, require you to show your ability to gather health and exercise history information, use interviews and questionnaires, and assess clients' current physical capabilities, attitudes, and goals for effective program design. For Domain II, Exercise Program Design and Implementation, examinees must be able to interpret the results of assessments to design exercise programs for clients based on their goals. Review the FITTE principle to prepare for this section of the test. Questions may ask about training methods, periodization, biomechanics, establishing and monitoring exercise intensity, program design for special populations, modifications, and other issues. You may also encounter questions about safe training and spotting practices, and signs of contraindications. For Exercise Leadership and Client Education, Domain III, prepare to demonstrate your knowledge about communication, motivation, and client education. Finally, Domain IV, Legal, Professional, Business, and Marketing, covers topics including the use of ACSM guidelines to obtain medical clearance for exercise programs, risk management, scope of practice, working with healthcare professionals, the ACSM Code of Ethics, and business issues, among others.

Each multiple-choice question is worth one raw point. The total number of questions you answer correctly is added up to obtain your raw score, which is then converted to a scale of 200 – 800. A passing score is 550 or higher. Scores are broken down by content area on score reports, so candidates can determine strengths and weaknesses. To register for an ACSM certification exam, visit the certification section on the ACSM website. This redirects to a separate page with additional information regarding the ACSM examination process and registration. The examination is taken either at a third-party certified testing center or at university testing centers. You will require a valid photo ID. ACSM members receive a discounted exam fee.

ONE: Practice Test One

_41

1. What is muscular hypertrophy?

A) an increase in the number of muscle cells

B) an increase in the size of the muscle cells

C) a decrease in the size of the muscle cells

D) an increase in the length of the muscle cells

2. Which assessment is used to determine upper body strength?

A) bench press test

B) push-up test

C) vertical jump test

D) barbell squat test

3. What muscular action occurs as a limb is pulled toward the midline of the body?

A) abduction

B) extension

C) pronation

D) adduction

4. An Olympic weightlifter who attempts a single repetition of an exercise for competition would benefit most from having which type of muscle?

A) type IIa

B) type I

C) slow-twitch

D) type IIb

5. Muscular atrophy occurs as a result of

A) performing the same exercises every workout.

B) lack of exercise or injury.

C) progressively overloading the muscles with a well-developed exercise program.

D) cardiovascular training.

6. Deficiencies of which vitamins or minerals can cause megaloblastic anemia?

A) thiamine

B) folate and vitamin B-12

C) iron

D) copper

7. What is the difference between a macromineral and a micromineral?

A) Macrominerals are larger than microminerals.

B) Macrominerals are required in the diet in larger quantities than microminerals.

C) Macrominerals bind together to from large complexes.

D) Microminerals are derived from microbial organisms in the gut.

8. During a gait assessment, the personal trainer should use the lateral view to check which kinetic chain checkpoint?

A) lumbo/pelvic/hip complex

B) head, low back, and shoulders

C) knees

D) ankles/feet

9. High blood LDL cholesterol is detrimental to cardiovascular health; soluble fiber can lower LDL cholesterol levels. Which of the following foods contain soluble fiber?

A) oatmeal, fruits, and beans

B) meat and dairy products

C) whole wheat, brown rice, and seeds

D) vegetable oils

10. Which joint allows for the most freedom of movement?

A) ball-and-socket

B) hinge

C) saddle

D) uniaxial

11. How much time should an American adult commit to exercise each week?

A) 6.5 hours

B) 4.5 hours

C) 2.5 hours

D) 1.5 hours

12. What is the single-leg squat test used to assess?

A) muscular endurance

B) cardiorespiratory fitness

C) single-leg functional strength

D) bilateral lower body strength

13. Which of the following assessments measures muscular endurance?

A) push-up test

B) three-minute step test

C) overhead squat

D) barbell squat test

14. To ensure accuracy of the results, the resting heart rate should be taken at what time of the day?

A) before a workout

B) at the end of the work day

C) upon rising in the morning

D) while resting during a workout

15. Which of the following techniques is NOT used to assess body composition?

A) body mass index (BMI)

B) the Margaria-Kalamen test

C) bioelectrical impedance

D) dual-energy x-ray absorptiometry (DEXA)

16. What term describes the reason somebody does something?

    (A) motivation
    B) locus of control
    C) objective
    D) joy

17. What happens to a person's base of support when the feet are spread apart further?

    A) The base of support decreases.
    B) The base of support stays the same.
    C) Base of support is not related to a person's stance.
    (D) The base of support increases.

18. Which of the following is generally NOT part of a fitness assessment?

    A) flexibility assessment
    B) static posture assessment
    (C) daily caloric intake assessment
    D) cardiorespiratory capacity assessment

19. Which of the following components of fitness assessment is the best predictor of mortality?

    (A) cardiorespiratory fitness
    B) flexibility
    C) muscular power
    D) static posture

20. Unless given permission, a trainer should not post _____ or _____ _____ on social media sites.

    (A) contracts, medical disclosures
    B) pictures, client reviews
    C) client reviews, PAR-Q forms
    D) information about friends, family members

21. When taking a circumference measurement of the thigh, where should the tape measure be positioned?

    A) directly above the patella
    (B) eight inches above the patella
    C) ten inches above the patella
    D) at the smallest point of the upper leg

22. Which of the following is the strongest indicator of how a client's cardiorespiratory system is responding and adapting to exercise?

    (A) resting heart rate
    B) 1.5-mile run
    C) body composition
    D) muscular strength test

23. Which exercise can improve bone mineral density?

    A) non-impact exercise
    B) swimming
    (C) axial loading of the skeleton through weightlifting
    D) walking outside

24. Which questionnaire identifies injury or previous surgery?

    A) lifestyle
    B) PAR-Q
    (C) medical history
    D) general health history

25. During exercise that lasts over one hour, how much fluid intake is recommended to maintain hydration?

    (A) 20 – 36 oz. per hour
    B) 8 – 12 oz. per hour
    C) 10 – 15 oz. per hour
    D) 40 – 45 oz. per hour

26. What is the strongest predictor of exercise program adherence?

    A) goals

    B) body composition

    C) previous injury history

    D) exercise history

27. What is multiple sclerosis?

    A) a disease associated with memory loss and dementia that occurs later in life

    B) a disease affecting bone mineral density

    C) a disease that affects the myelin sheaths that surround axons on a neuron

    D) a disease that damages the nucleus of neurons

28. Body composition in relation to a healthy weight

    A) is a measure of the relative proportions of carbohydrates, proteins, fat, and water in the body.

    B) is the percentage of fat-free mass versus fat mass in the body.

    C) is the percentage of bone versus soft tissue in the body.

    D) is the percentage of dry mass versus water in the body.

29. Which macronutrients are the major fuels for exercise?

    A) carbohydrates and fats

    B) protein and carbohydrates

    C) protein and fats

    D) carbohydrates, fats, and protein

30. During the overhead squat assessment, the personal trainer observes flattening of the feet. Which of the following terms describes what the personal trainer is observing?

    A) posterior pelvic tilt

    B) lower crossed syndrome

    C) pronation distortion syndrome

    D) upper crossed syndrome

31. How long should the rest period be between sets of deadlifts at five repetitions and heavy loads?

    A) one minute

    B) less than thirty seconds

    C) three minutes

    D) six minutes

32. How can a trainer tell if the client is legitimately at an eight or nine on the RPE scale?

    A) The client will tell the trainer.

    B) The client will be unable to complete sentences since the client will be breathing so heavily.

    C) The trainer will not be able to tell.

    D) The client will be able to speak full sentences describing the intensity.

33. Which of the following is NOT a benefit of exercise testing?

    A) assessing physical work capacity

    B) assessing movement capabilities

    C) determining if a medical referral will be needed prior to exercise

    D) determining acute variables for an exercise program

34. For a test to be valid, it must be
    A) reliable.
    B) helpful.
    C) difficult.
    D) easy.

35. What type of training uses controlled instability to increase proprioception?
    A) plyometrics
    B) cardio training
    C) free weight training
    D) core training

36. A lifestyle questionnaire should NOT include questions which pertain to which of the following?
    A) sleep
    B) stress
    C) friends
    D) smoking

37. Which of the following will give the personal trainer a general idea of an individual's movement foundation?
    A) dynamic movement
    B) flexibility
    C) static posture
    D) proprioception

38. A static postural assessment will provide information on the following, EXCEPT
    A) proper cardiovascular function.
    B) joint misalignment.
    C) proper muscle length.
    D) possible muscular dysfunction.

39. Which postural misalignment is characterized by rounded shoulders and a forward head position?
    A) lower crossed syndrome
    B) upper crossed syndrome
    C) pronation distortion
    D) knee valgus

40. Which of the following refers to the degree to which a test or test item measures what is supposed to be measured?
    A) relativity
    B) honesty
    C) validity
    D) strength

41. Which of the following tests is used to estimate aerobic capacity (VO2 max)?
    A) three-minute step
    B) Margaria-Kalamen
    C) Rockport walk
    D) 300-yard shuttle

42. Proper breathing technique controls
    A) power, stabilization, and strength.
    B) core activation, repetition tempo, and range of motion.
    C) caloric expenditure, power, and range of motion.
    D) core activation, power, and mind.

43. During the three-minute step test, the metronome should be set to how many beats per minute?
    A) ninety
    B) eighty-two
    C) ninety-six
    D) one hundred and six

44. A foam roller is used for what type of training?

- **A)** PNF stretching
- **B)** active stretching
- **C)** power training
- **D)** self-myofascial release

45. Advanced lifters who are lifting heavy loads adopt which type of breathing technique?

- **A)** Valsalva Breathing Maneuver
- **B)** Pierogi Breath Training
- **C)** Concentric/Eccentric Breathing Technique
- **D)** Power and Stability Breathing Maneuver

46. Ligaments adhere

- **A)** bone to bone.
- **B)** bone to muscle.
- **C)** muscle to muscle.
- **D)** cartilage to bone.

47. Which test is most suitable to assess lower body strength?

- **A)** long jump
- **B)** barbell squat
- **C)** overhead squat
- **D)** hexagon

48. In a standing or sitting position, a client should maintain which three points of contact?

- **A)** shoulders, calves, heels
- **B)** head, shoulders, glutes
- **C)** head, glutes, calves
- **D)** shoulders, glutes, heels

49. What are open kinetic chain exercises?

- **A)** exercises that allow foot or hand movement
- **B)** exercises that load the spine
- **C)** exercises that keep either feet or hands at a fixed point
- **D)** exercises that rely on a partner to stretch the limbs

50. Which of the following skinfold sites is used when performing a three-site skinfold equation for a fifty-two-year-old woman?

- **A)** chest
- **B)** abdomen
- **C)** thigh
- **D)** subscapular

51. The sit-and-reach test is used to measure the flexibility of which of the following muscles?

- **A)** shoulders and upper back
- **B)** shoulders and lower back
- **C)** quadriceps and lower back
- **D)** lower back and hamstring

52. Which of these refers to a muscular contraction during which the muscle resists a force as it lengthens?

- **A)** eccentric muscle contraction
- **B)** concentric muscle contraction
- **C)** isotonic muscle contraction
- **D)** isometric muscle contraction

53. Assisted stretching is also known as _____.

- **A)** SMR
- **B)** foam rolling
- **C)** dynamic
- **D)** PNF

54. If the rest period is around thirty seconds and the load is light, which repetition range is most appropriate?

   A) one repetition
   B) eight repetitions
   C) ten repetitions
   D) fifteen repetitions

55. An effective warm-up should last between 5 – 10 minutes at what type of intensity?

   A) moderate to high intensity
   B) multiple interval intensity
   C) low to moderate intensity
   D) high intensity

56. Which of the following exercise deterrents is NOT an environmental factor?

   A) gender
   B) time
   C) weather
   D) social support

57. Which of the following is NOT among HIPAA's primary objectives?

   A) to simplify obtaining and keeping health insurance
   B) to protect school records
   C) to protect the privacy and security of healthcare information
   D) to aid the healthcare industry in streamlining and minimizing administrative costs

58. When spotting a shoulder press, where should the spotter's hands be?

   A) wrists
   B) elbows
   C) neck
   D) back

59. What types of exercises are considered dynamic stretches?

   A) med ball chops and prisoner squats
   B) barbell deadlifts and arm circles
   C) butt kickers and hamstring static stretch
   D) squat jumps and shoulder push press

60. An effective cooldown

   A) should mimic the warm-up to ensure steady heart rate reduction.
   B) should start with falling on the floor in exhaustion.
   C) should still have weight training in it.
   D) should have the client just walking around.

61. If the client has potentially harmful health issues during an initial meeting to discuss a fitness program, the trainer should

   A) advise the client to visit a physician for medical clearance to exercise.
   B) take the client's word on whether they are healthy enough for exercise.
   C) ignore the health concern until it comes up during the course of the program.
   D) send the client to a manager to train.

62. In the power phase of fitness training, what is the primary training emphasis?

   A) improving muscle endurance
   B) building prime mover strength
   C) muscle speed and force production
   D) balance training

63. Which is an alternative to standard aerobic training?

    A) plyometrics
    B) stretching
    C) core training
    D) circuit training

64. Which behavior change model focuses on understanding the relationship between a person and his or her environment?

    A) readiness-to-change model
    B) social cognitive theory model
    C) theory of planned behavior
    D) socio-ecological model

65. What is a regression of a kettlebell swing?

    A) straight leg deadlift
    B) box jump
    C) single-arm swing
    D) front raise

66. What is the primary mover for a wrist curl?

    A) triceps
    B) forearm
    C) shoulder
    D) biceps

67. What is a regression for a push press?

    A) seated dumbbell shoulder press
    B) standing upright row
    C) low pulley row
    D) push-up

68. What are the three top accredited certifying agencies that set the standards of practice for the fitness industry?

    A) NASM, ACE, and ISSA
    B) NASM, ACE, and ACSM
    C) NCCA, ANSI, and ISSA
    D) ACSM, NSCA, and ACE

69. Inconsistency of a muscle around a joint is considered a

    _____.

    A) muscle knot
    B) muscle imbalance
    C) muscle explosion
    D) muscle structure

70. A floor crunch is a regression for what core exercise?

    A) reverse crunch
    B) plank hold
    C) hip bridge
    D) ball crunch

71. A grip used primarily in parallel bar or dumbbell pushing and pulling movements where the thumbs stay up and the palms face each other is:

    A) supinated grip
    B) alternating grip
    C) false grip
    D) neutral grip

72. The allied healthcare continuum (AHC) includes all the following professionals, EXCEPT

    A) a nurse.
    B) a psychologist.
    C) an occupational therapist.
    D) a psychic.

73. Which exercise is most beneficial for basketball players' peak performance?

   A) bench press

   B) leg press

   C) squat jumps

   D) rotator cuff exercises

74. What is a regression for a ball crunch?

   A) single leg windmill

   B) bent leg sit-up

   C) abdominal crunch

   D) cable rotation

75. Based on the principle of specificity, the fact that football players run one hundred yards at most should tell the trainer not to implement

   A) short-distance sprint intervals in the training program.

   B) long-distance running into the training program.

   C) power exercises for improved speed in the training program.

   D) muscular endurance exercises into the training program.

76. Performing a specific number of repetitions through the full range of motion is called

   A) a workout.

   B) the load.

   C) overload.

   D) a set.

77. Rest period refers to the break during workouts between which two of the following?

   A) sets and progressions

   B) sets and exercises

   C) sets and range of motion

   D) strength and endurance

78. Detraining occurs more rapidly

   A) in cardiovascular health.

   B) in muscular strength.

   C) in clients who have previously trained.

   D) in professional athletes.

79. When should a personal trainer terminate a cardiorespiratory assessment?

   A) when the client's heart rate increases

   B) when the client requests to stop

   C) when the client begins to perspire

   D) when the client begins to fatigue

80. Which of the following is most likely to cause a muscular imbalance of the upper body?

   A) a training program that utilizes alternating push and pull exercises

   B) a bodyweight training program that includes exercises for the chest, back, core, and legs

   C) a well-balanced yoga routine with a trained instructor

   D) a unilateral training program emphasizing strengthening of the pectorals and anterior deltoids

81. Resistance training programs for children and adolescents should focus on

   A) increasing weight lifted.

   B) specific and repetitive movements.

   C) high-intensity exercise.

   D) proper technique and form.

82. Which grip is overhanded?

   A) alternated grip

   B) supinated grip

   C) pronated grip

   D) clean grip

83. Which two might be the proper regression and progression of the push-up exercise?

   A) alternating single-leg push-ups and BOSU Ball push-ups

   B) push-ups with feet elevated and clapping push-ups

   C) kneeling push-ups and wall push-ups (hands on wall)

   D) kneeling push-ups and push-ups with feet elevated

84. Which test would be the most important indicator of a client's ability to complete the activities of daily living?

   A) strength test

   B) cardiorespiratory test

   C) movement test

   D) static posture test

85. Which answer describes why the following is not a SMART goal?

   The client wants to lose twenty-five pounds in two months.

   A) The goal is not specific.

   B) The goal is not time-stamped.

   C) The goal is not realistic.

   D) The goal is not measurable.

86. If a client has had a recent joint surgery, what should the trainer do before starting the fitness program?

   A) a fitness assessment

   B) require the client to get a physician's clearance to exercise

   C) take the client through a workout and avoid the injured joint

   D) tell the client to work out on his own

87. When should PNF stretching be implemented into the program?

   A) during the warm-up

   B) during the resistance training phase

   C) before performing cardiovascular exercise

   D) during the flexibility and cooldown

88. Novice clients' rest periods may differ from those of advanced clients in that

   A) novices will require less rest before starting the next set of an exercise.

   B) novices may require more rest periods per workout than advanced clients.

   C) novices should get rest periods only between different exercises but not between sets.

   D) novices should get rest periods only between sets but not between exercises.

89. Along with proper body positioning, another way to isolate muscle groups with efficiency is to use different types of _____ while lifting barbells, dumbbells, or kettlebells, and while using weight machines.

   A) weights

   B) breathing

   C) grips

   D) swings

90. The Karvonen formula is used to calculate

   A) maximum heart rate.

   B) target heart rate.

   C) resting heart rate.

   D) heart rate recovery.

91. The 1RM test measures the client's

A) ability to perform an exercise at the maximal effort of strength for a single repetition.

B) weight utilized for all exercises in the program.

C) target heart rate zone.

D) ability to perform an exercise at submaximal efforts for multiple repetitions.

92. Which of the following tests determines an exercise program's progression or regression?

A) pretest

B) midtest

C) post-test

D) formative evaluation

93. Which two effects of cardiovascular training are consistent between aerobic and anaerobic exercise during the workout?

A) increased heart rate and lactate threshold

B) increased heart rate and type II muscle fiber recruitment

C) increased heart rate and respiration rate

D) increased blood pressure and type I muscle fiber recruitment

94. CEC stands for

A) constant educational content.

B) continuing education credit.

C) collective exercise collaboration.

D) care education collective.

95. The second transition period is a period of

A) high-intensity training.

B) sports-specific training.

C) no physical activity at all.

D) active recovery involving non-specific recreational activity.

96. A superset in a training program refers to

A) performing an exercise and gradually increasing load, then decreasing load per set.

B) performing multiple sets of a single exercise with intermittent rest periods.

C) performing an exercise and then immediately performing another exercise utilizing the antagonist or opposite muscle groups.

D) performing a series of different exercises in a row with a rest period at the end of the series.

97. Self-efficacy is

A) self-control.

B) willpower.

C) self-love.

D) belief in oneself.

98. Program design for athletic improvement relies heavily on

A) exercise specificity.

B) resistance training every day.

C) cardiovascular training every day.

D) the amount of weight the athlete can lift for one repetition.

99. Injury is categorized as which type of barrier to exercise adherence?

   A) environmental factor

   B) personal attribute

   C) physical-activity factor

   D) locus of control

100. The steady progression of microcycles from muscular endurance to hypertrophy, to strength, and finally to power, describes what type of periodization?

   A) undulating periodization

   B) recreational periodization

   C) linear periodization

   D) sports-specific periodization

101. The repetition range for development of muscular hypertrophy is between

   A) one and five repetitions.

   B) fifteen and twenty repetitions.

   C) ten and fifteen repetitions.

   D) eight and twelve repetitions.

102. The learning stage of progression associated with the client mastering an exercise technique without movement compensations is

   A) the autonomous stage.

   B) the cognitive stage.

   C) the continual stage.

   D) the associative stage.

103. Which test is used to measure maximal speed?

   A) forty-yard dash

   B) three-hundred-yard shuttle

   C) 1.5-mile run

   D) pro-shuttle

104. How should the trainer modify abdominal exercises, such as the crunch, for pregnant clients?

   A) No modification is necessary.

   B) Reduce the range of motion dramatically.

   C) Pregnant clients are not allowed to perform abdominal exercises.

   D) Have the client seated slightly upright.

105. Income is categorized as which type of barrier to exercise adherence?

   A) personal attribute

   B) environmental factor

   C) physical-activity factor

   D) core factor

106. Detraining occurs more quickly in

   A) resistance training gains.

   B) cardiovascular training gains.

   C) men.

   D) women.

107. What should be done in addition to dynamic stretching during the warm-up process?

   A) light to moderate cardiovascular exercise

   B) plyometric exercises

   C) agility exercises

   D) resistance training

108. Employing a personal trainer because someone wants to fit in a size six wedding dress would be considered what?

   A) vain

   B) intrinsically motivated

   C) obese

   D) extrinsically motivated

109. One major advantage of zone training in cardiovascular exercise programs is that

  A) it is always low intensity and safe.

  B) the mode does not change so it is easy to remember.

  C) it provides variety in cardiovascular training, which helps with program compliance.

  D) it takes less time than steady-state aerobic training.

110. Program design for senior citizens should incorporate exercises that improve

  A) muscular power.

  B) the ability to perform daily tasks.

  C) anaerobic endurance.

  D) arm strength.

111. People who believe that life is controlled by things that happen to them have _____ locus of control.

  A) an internal

  B) an intrinsic

  C) an external

  D) a skewed

112. How many American adults get the minimum recommended levels of activity, according to the CDC?

  A) 20 percent

  B) 75 percent

  C) 45 percent

  D) 90 percent

113. All these are more advanced forms of aerobic training EXCEPT

  A) jumping rope.

  B) rowing machine.

  C) walking.

  D) running.

114. _____ can be considered the most difficult of exercise adherence barriers to overcome.

  A) Income and fitness level

  B) Accessibility and self-efficacy

  C) Locus of control and intrinsic motivators

  D) Self-efficacy and locus of control

115. Improving lactate threshold can be accomplished by the trainer implementing

  A) steady-state cardiovascular training.

  B) maximal-strength resistance training.

  C) muscular power training.

  D) sprint interval training.

116. According to the CDC, thirty-four percent of adults in the US are

  A) overweight.

  B) morbidly obese.

  C) a healthy weight.

  D) obese.

117. Where should the rules and regulations for an emergency action plan be obtained?

  A) from fitness websites

  B) from certified fitness professionals

  C) from the US Department of Labor

  D) from any local business

118. Among individuals adhering to a fitness program, 50 percent of them drop out after:

  A) three weeks

  B) two months

  C) six months

  D) eight months

119. Personal attributes, which can hinder exercise adherence, include all of the following, EXCEPT what?

   A) age
   B) accessibility
   C) time
   D) fitness level

120. Which term describes using specific movements or words to inform participants of upcoming events?

   A) cueing
   B) exercise
   C) phrasing
   D) sign language

121. Fitness professionals should keep clients' emergency contact information

   A) stored in their cell phones.
   B) on an email list.
   C) filed on the work computer.
   D) alphabetized in a locked, easily accessible filing cabinet.

122. In the _____ phase of change, the individual has taken definitive steps to change his or her behavior.

   A) precontemplation
   B) maintenance
   C) action
   D) preparation

123. Because of an increased Q-angle, female athletes are at a higher risk of medial knee injuries in which sport(s)?

   A) rock climbing
   B) basketball and volleyball
   C) ice hockey
   D) snowboarding

124. Which of the following is NOT among the ways personal trainers can earn CECs?

   A) college courses
   B) industry specialization certification
   C) blog contributions
   D) structured learning modules from accredited programs

125. A trainer who provides advice or information beyond a certified or licensed specialty is working outside of the

   A) mode of specialty.
   B) gym walls.
   C) scope of practice.
   D) health profession.

126. Which term describes positive feedback emphasizing a specific aspect of an individual's behavior or task?

   A) kinesthetic feedback
   B) positive reinforcement
   C) targeted praise
   D) non-verbal communication

127. Miscellaneous personal trainer's insurance covers which type of claims?

   A) defamation
   B) wrongful invasion of privacy
   C) wrongful termination
   D) bodily injury

128. When someone initiates a plan to solve a problem within a month, that person is in the _____ phase.

   A) preparation
   B) contemplation
   C) action
   D) termination

129. What does READ stand for?

A) rapport, enthusiasm, antecedent, determine

B) reinforce, empathy, approve, decide

C) rapport, entertain, assessment, decide

D) rapport, empathy, assessment, development

130. Which of the following is an organ associated with controlling the release of chemical substances, known as hormones, for the regulation of metabolic processes, growth, development, sexual reproduction, and other bodily functions?

A) a hormone

B) the brain

C) testosterone

D) a gland

131. Anabolic steroid abuse can cause

A) brain damage.

B) memory loss.

C) liver damage.

D) muscular atrophy.

132. What is one method for signaling and alerting emergency authorities?

A) setting off a fire alarm

B) shouting for help

C) calling a friend

D) emailing an authority figure

133. Which exercise might be implemented in the first transition period of a triathlete's fitness program?

A) alternating leg bounding plyometrics

B) a standard wall sit

C) barbell bench press

D) tricep kickbacks

134. The RICE acronym should be followed when a person has

A) injuries involving severe bleeding.

B) injuries involving sprains, strains, or contusions.

C) injuries involving cardiopulmonary issues.

D) injuries involving chest pain.

135. What is voluntary commitment to an exercise program known as?

A) exercise selection

B) motivation

C) exercise adherence

D) exercise commitment

136. If a client appears to have mastered the exercise in a workout, the trainer should

A) implement a progression of the exercise the client mastered.

B) implement a regression of the exercise the client mastered.

C) stop the client from exercising.

D) implement a totally new workout.

137. Which of the following is a glucose-based energy supply that is typically synthesized and stored in the liver and skeletal muscle of the human body?

A) blood sugar

B) acetyl CoA

C) creatine phosphate

D) glycogen

138. Income can be categorized as a(n) _____ _____ barrier to exercise adherence and motivation.

A) environmental factor

B) personal attribute

C) self-efficacy

D) physical-activity factor

139. Performing a calf raise is an example of which type of lever?

A) a first-class lever

B) It is not a type of lever.

C) a second-class lever

D) a third-class lever

140. Monitoring exercise intensity is a means of

A) making workouts more fun for clients.

B) making sure everyone is exercising at the same pace.

C) making sure the client gets good value from the training sessions.

D) reducing the risks involved with exercise.

141. Movement assessments are used to test

A) maximal force.

B) core strength.

C) agility and speed.

D) dynamic posture.

142. Which planning step uses measurable goals to aid the trainer in determining whether a client is getting closer to meeting his or her long-term goals?

A) belief

B) vision

C) learning

D) persistence

143. Which statement does NOT outline a proper security procedure for protecting confidential client information on a computer or other electronic device?

A) be sure all computers and electronic devices are password protected

B) be sure all computers and electronic devices have anti-virus protection

C) be sure all computers and electronic devices are easily accessible to employees

D) be sure all computers and electronic devices have malware protection software

144. Regardless of whether a fitness professional is considered a gym employee, all trainers should obtain what?

A) liability insurance

B) a group fitness certification

C) fitness equipment

D) a social media account

145. Personal trainers obtain what type of information from their clients in the first meeting?

A) gossip

B) sensitive

C) humorous

D) basic

146. A false grip is

    A)   an underhanded grip.

    B)   where the thumb is wrapped around the bar along with the fingers.

    C)   where the thumb is wrapped around the bar on the opposite side of the fingers.

    D)   where the thumb is facing the ceiling and the palms are toward the body.

147. Which machines use a combination of the body's concentric and eccentric force, gravity, and the friction from the pulleys and weight loaded to dictate the speed of the machine and range of motion?

    A)   free weights

    B)   hydraulic machines

    C)   suspension trainers

    D)   cam machines

148. Which of the following is NOT a potential risk factor associated with clients requiring medical clearance?

    A)   sedentary lifestyle

    B)   high blood pressure

    C)   low resting heart rate

    D)   obesity

149. Basic Life Support (BLS) certification courses for fitness professionals should include training in

    A)   CPR only.

    B)   AED only.

    C)   first aid, CPR, and AED.

    D)   evaluating cardiac arrhythmias.

150. Some personal trainers provide _____ advice, which can fall outside of their scope of practice unless they are further certified.

    A)   exercise

    B)   stretching

    C)   general health

    D)   nutrition

1. A) Incorrect. This refers to hyperplasia.

    B) Correct. This is the definition of muscular hypertrophy.

    C) Incorrect. This refers to muscular atrophy.

    D) Incorrect. This is not the definition of muscular hypertrophy.

2. **A) Correct.** The bench press test is used to determine upper body strength.

    B) Incorrect. The push-up test is used to assess muscular endurance.

    C) Incorrect. The vertical jump test is used to measure lower body explosiveness.

    D) Incorrect. The barbell squat test is used to measure lower body strength.

3. A) Incorrect. This occurs when a limb is pulled away from the midline of the body.

    B) Incorrect. This occurs as a joint angle increases with muscle contraction.

    C) Incorrect. This occurs as the hand is rotated so the palm faces toward the ground.

    D) Correct. This muscular action refers to adduction.

4. A) Incorrect. Type IIb muscles are more beneficial.

    B) Incorrect. Type I muscle would not provide much benefit.

    C) Incorrect. Slow-twitch fibers are the same as type I and won't benefit the lifter much.

    D) Correct. Olympic weightlifters benefit most from having type IIb muscle fibers for maximal power output.

5. A) Incorrect. This will not induce muscular atrophy.

    B) Correct. Lack of exercise or injury can cause muscular atrophy.

    C) Incorrect. This will induce the opposite, known as muscular hypertrophy.

    D) Incorrect. This will not cause muscular atrophy.

6. A) Incorrect. Thiamine plays no role in anemia.

    B) Correct. Folate and vitamin B-12 are critical to the synthesis of nucleotides, which are the building blocks of DNA. When DNA synthesis is impaired, red blood cells cannot divide fast enough and instead grow large.

    C) Incorrect. The type of anemia caused by iron deficiency is characterized by a lack of hemoglobin, which is needed to carry sufficient oxygen.

    D) Incorrect. Copper deficiency can lead to iron-deficiency anemia because it is involved in iron transport, not megaloblastic anemia.

7. A) Incorrect. The size of the mineral atom has nothing to do with the naming.

    B) Correct. Macrominerals are typically present in the body in larger quantities and have larger dietary requirements.

    C) Incorrect. Macrominerals do not bind together.

    D) Incorrect. Minerals are obtained from the diet.

8. A) Incorrect. The LPHC should be viewed posteriorly.

    B) Correct. These checkpoints should be viewed laterally.

    C) Incorrect. The knees should be viewed anteriorly.

    D) Incorrect. The ankles and feet should be viewed anteriorly.

9. **A) Correct.** Oatmeal, fruits, and beans are sources of soluble fiber.

    B) Incorrect. Only plant foods contain fiber.

    C) Incorrect. Whole wheat, brown rice, and seeds are sources of insoluble fiber.

    D) Incorrect. Vegetable oils contain only fats.

10. **A) Correct.** Ball-and-socket joints allow for the most freedom of movement.

B) Incorrect. Hinge joints only allow for flexion and extension.

C) Incorrect. Saddle joints do not allow rotation.

D) Incorrect. Uniaxial joints only allow for movement through one plane of motion.

11. A) Incorrect. Exercising for 6.5 hours each week is above the recommended amount.

B) Incorrect. Committing 4.5 hours each week to exercise is above the recommended amount.

C) **Correct.** A weekly total of 2.5 hours is the standard amount of exercise recommended.

D) Incorrect. A total of 1.5 hours is below the recommended amount for exercise each week.

12. A) Incorrect. The repetitions of the test are not enough to assess muscular endurance.

B) Incorrect. The single-leg squat does not assess cardiorespiratory fitness.

C) **Correct.** One of the components the single-leg squat test measures is single-leg strength.

D) Incorrect. The single-leg squat test measures unilateral leg strength.

13. A) **Correct.** The push-up test is used to assess the stability of the muscular endurance of the upper body.

B) Incorrect. The three-minute step test is a cardiorespiratory assessment.

C) Incorrect. The overhead squat test is used to assess dynamic movement and flexibility.

D) Incorrect. The barbell squat test is used to assess lower body strength.

14. A) Incorrect. A heart rate taken before a workout would be considered a preworkout heart rate.

B) Incorrect. A heart rate taken at the end of the day may be affected by factors such as stress, food, or beverages consumed.

C) **Correct.** The best time to measure resting heart rate is upon rising in the morning for three consecutive days.

D) Incorrect. Taking heart rate measurements during a workout would alter the heart rate due to the activity level.

15. A) Incorrect. Body mass index measurements are used to assess body composition.

B) **Correct.** The Margaria-Kalamen test is used to assess muscular power.

C) Incorrect. Bioelectrical impedance is a method used to assess body composition.

D) Incorrect. The DEXA scan is used to assess body composition.

16. A) **Correct.** Motivation is the reason why somebody does something.

B) Incorrect. Locus of control is a factor in adherence to goals.

C) Incorrect. Objectives are considered goals, and motivation will keep a person focused on those goals.

D) Incorrect. Joy is an emotion possibly felt after achieving goals.

17. A) Incorrect. The base of support decreases when the feet are closer together.

B) Incorrect. Stance width changes the base of support.

C) Incorrect. The base of support is directly related to stance.

D) **Correct.** The base of support increases with a wider foot stance.

18. A) Incorrect. A flexibility assessment is generally included in a fitness assessment.

B) Incorrect. A static postural assessment is generally included in a fitness assessment.

C) **Correct.** An assessment of daily caloric intake is generally not included during a fitness assessment.

D) Incorrect. A cardiorespiratory capacity assessment is generally not included in a fitness assessment.

19. **A) Correct.** Cardiorespiratory fitness would be the most accurate predictor of mortality due to its stressing of the heart, veins, and arteries.

    B) Incorrect. Flexibility would not be a predictor of mortality.

    C. Incorrect. Muscular power is not the best indicator of mortality.

    D. Incorrect. Static posture would not be the best indicator of mortality.

20. A) Incorrect. Information such as contracts and medical disclosures should NEVER be posted or shared.

    B) Correct. Pictures and client reviews may be posted on social media to promote a trainer, as long as the client gives permission.

    C) Incorrect. Client reviews and PAR-Q forms should NEVER be posted online.

    D) Incorrect. Posting personal or family information puts a trainer's privacy at risk.

21. A) Incorrect. Placing the tape measure directly above the patella would not provide a measurement of the girth of the leg.

    B) Incorrect. Placing the tape measure eight inches above the patella is not the correct position.

    C) Correct. The tape measure should be placed ten inches above the patella.

    D) Incorrect. The tape measure should be placed around the widest point of the upper leg.

22. **A) Correct.** The resting heart rate is the strongest indicator of how the cardiorespiratory system is responding and adapting to exercise.

    B) Incorrect. The 1.5-mile run is an assessment of cardiorespiratory fitness but does not provide a strong indicator of how the cardiorespiratory system responds to exercise.

C) Incorrect. Body composition is not an indicator of cardiorespiratory fitness.

D) Incorrect. Muscular strength is not an indicator of cardiorespiratory fitness.

23. A) Incorrect. Non-impact exercise does not load the skeleton to elicit improvement to bone mineral density.

    B) Incorrect. Swimming is a form of non-impact exercise.

    C) Correct. Axial loading of the skeleton through weight lifting improves and maintains bone mineral density.

    D) Incorrect. Though walking does involve impact, it is a relatively low-impact exercise.

24. A) Incorrect. The lifestyle questionnaire identifies lifestyle habits.

    B) Incorrect. The PAR-Q helps identify a client's readiness for an exercise program.

    C) Correct. A medical history questionnaire provides information regarding any past injuries or surgeries.

    D) Incorrect. A general health history questionnaire may not provide details about previous surgeries.

25. **A) Correct.** To maintain hydration, it is recommended to consume 20 – 36 oz. of fluid, preferably a sport drink with electrolytes, and ideally spread out at 15 – 20 minute intervals.

    B) Incorrect. A fluid intake of 8 – 12 oz. per hour is not enough to maintain hydration during periods of prolonged exercise.

    C) Incorrect. A fluid intake of 10 – 15 oz. per hour is not enough to maintain hydration during prolonged exercise.

    D) Incorrect. It would be difficult to consume 40 – 45 oz. of fluid per hour, and such a quantity is more than necessary to maintain hydration.

26. A) Incorrect. Client goals will not predict exercise program adherence.

    B) Incorrect. Body composition is not a predictor of exercise program adherence.

C) Incorrect. Previous injury history could be a predictor of exercise program adherence but is not the strongest.

D) Correct. Exercise history is the strongest predictor of exercise program adherence since it will detail previous exercise habits.

27. A) Incorrect. This refers to Alzheimer's disease.

B) Incorrect. This refers to osteoporosis.

C) Correct. Multiple sclerosis affects the myelin sheaths on axons.

D) Incorrect. Multiple sclerosis affects the myelin sheaths rather than the nucleus.

28. A) Incorrect. Body composition does not divide out carbohydrates, protein, or water.

B) Correct. Body composition refers to the relative percentage of fat versus everything else: muscle, soft tissues, organs, and bone.

C) Incorrect. Both bone and soft tissues contribute to fat-free mass.

D) Incorrect. There is water associated with both the fat mass and fat-free mass.

29. **A) Correct.** Carbohydrates in the form of muscle glycogen and possibly liver glycogen, along with blood glucose, muscle triglycerides, blood fatty acids, and lipoproteins are the major fuels for exercise.

B) Incorrect. Although protein can provide fuel for exercise, its contribution is minor compared to that of carbohydrates and fat.

C) Incorrect. Contributions from protein to fuel exercise are minor compared to the contributions made by carbohydrates.

D) Incorrect. The contributions proteins make to fueling exercise are minor; carbohydrates and fat are the main fuels for exercise.

30. A) Incorrect. Posterior pelvic tilt is characterized by a posterior tilt of the pelvis.

B) Incorrect. Lower crossed syndrome is characterized by an anterior tilt of the pelvis.

C) Correct. One of the characteristics of pronation distortion syndrome is flattening of the feet.

D) Incorrect. Upper crossed syndrome is characterized by a forward head position and rounded shoulders.

31. A) Incorrect. A one-minute rest period is insufficient for recovery.

B) Incorrect. A rest period of less than thirty seconds is far too short for recovery.

C) Correct. At heavy loads and low volumes, rest periods should be three minutes.

D) Incorrect. Six minutes is too long a recovery period, and the muscles will start to cool down.

32. A) Incorrect. The client and the trainer may have different perceptions of an eight or nine on the scale.

B) Correct. The client will not be able to complete sentences because the intensity will be so high.

C) Incorrect. The trainer should be able to distinguish how difficult an exercise is for the client using the RPE scale along with other methods of measuring intensity.

D) Incorrect. At this intensity, the client will likely not be able to complete sentences between breaths.

33. A) Incorrect. Exercise testing will measure physical work capacity.

B) Incorrect. Exercise testing will assess movement capabilities.

C) Correct. The initial interview will determine if a medical referral is needed, not exercise testing.

D) Incorrect. Exercise testing will help the personal trainer select the proper acute variables for the client's exercise program.

34. **A) Correct.** A test must be reliable for it to be valid.

B) Incorrect. This is not a requirement for a test to be valid.

C) Incorrect. This is not a requirement for a test to be valid.

D) Incorrect. This is not a requirement for a test to be valid.

35. A) Incorrect. Plyometrics training increases force production.

B) Incorrect. Cardio training increases aerobic endurance.

C) Incorrect. Free weight training increases prime mover and joint strength.

D) Correct. Core training increases core strength with balance.

36. A) Incorrect. Questions pertaining to a client's sleep patterns should be included on a lifestyle questionnaire.

B) Incorrect. Questions pertaining to a client's stressors should be included on a lifestyle questionnaire.

C) Correct. Questions pertaining to a client's friends are not necessary on a lifestyle questionnaire.

D) Incorrect. Questions pertaining to a client's smoking habits should be included on a lifestyle questionnaire.

37. A) Incorrect. This will give the trainer a general idea of an individual's range of motion.

B) Incorrect. This will give the trainer a general idea of an individual's muscle extensibility and joint mobility.

C) Correct. This will give the trainer a general idea of an individual's movement foundation.

D) Incorrect. This will give the trainer a general idea of an individual's ability to balance.

38. A) Correct. A static postural assessment cannot provide information about a client's heart health.

B) Incorrect. A static postural assessment can provide information about joint misalignment.

C) Incorrect. A static postural assessment can provide information about proper muscle length.

D) Incorrect. A static postural assessment can provide information about possible muscular dysfunction.

39. A) Incorrect. This is associated with misaligned lumbo/pelvic/hip complex.

B) Correct. This is associated with misaligned neck, shoulders, and midback.

C) Incorrect. This is associated with misalignment of the feet and ankles.

D) Incorrect. This is associated with pronation distortion, causing the knees to internally rotate.

40. A) Incorrect. Relativity refers to a theory in physics.

B) Incorrect. Honesty refers to the principle of personal values.

C) Correct. This term describes the degree to which a test or test item measures what is supposed to be measured.

D) Incorrect. This is part of an assessment.

41. A) Incorrect. This test is used to measure cardiorespiratory fitness and how quickly the heart rate recovers from short bouts of exercise.

B) Incorrect. This test is used to measure lower body power.

C) Correct. This test is used to measure VO2 max.

D) Incorrect. This test is used to measure anaerobic capacity.

42. A) Incorrect. Power, stabilization, and strength are phases of the training continuum.

B) Correct. Proper breathing technique controls core activation, repetition tempo, and range of motion.

C) Incorrect. This answer is only partially correct. Breathing technique controls range of motion, but it cannot control the body's caloric expenditure;

furthermore, *power* describes a phase in the training continuum.

D) Incorrect. This answer is only partially correct. Breathing technique controls core activation, but it cannot fully control the mind; furthermore, *power* describes a phase in the training continuum.

43. A) Incorrect. Ninety steps per minute would not complete the test.

B) Incorrect. Eighty-two steps per minute would not complete the test.

C) Correct. The metronome should be set to ninety-six beats per minute.

D) Incorrect. One hundred and six steps per minute would exceed the three-minute mark.

44. A) Incorrect. A stretching partner is used in PNF stretching.

B) Incorrect. Active stretching uses bodyweight only.

C) Incorrect. Boxes and medicine balls are used for power training.

D) Correct. SMR utilizes gravity and a foam roller to ease muscle tension.

45. **A) Correct.** The Valsalva Breathing Maneuver is a specific breathing technique used when a lifter is challenged with heavy loads.

B) Incorrect. A pierogi is a potato dumpling and has nothing to do with exercise.

C) Incorrect. The Concentric/Eccentric Breathing Technique is a generalized breathing technique that should be used whether one is lifting heavy loads or not and does not require the lifter to hold their breath.

D) Incorrect. The Power and Stability Breathing Maneuver is not an actual breathing technique.

46. **A) Correct.** Ligaments adhere bone to bone.

B) Incorrect. This refers to tendons.

C) Incorrect. This is not the function of ligaments.

D) Incorrect. This is not the function of ligaments.

47. A) Incorrect. The long jump test is used to measure maximal jumping distance.

B) Correct. The barbell squat test is used to measure lower body strength.

C) Incorrect. The overhead squat assesses dynamic flexibility.

D) Incorrect. The hexagon test is used to measure agility.

48. A) Incorrect. Only the shoulders are a point of contact in a standing or sitting position.

B) Correct. These are the three parts of the body that should maintain points of contact with the wall or dowel.

C) Incorrect. The calves are not a point of contact in a standing or sitting position.

D) Incorrect. The heels are not a point of contact in a standing or sitting position.

49. **A) Correct.** Exercises that allow foot or hand movement keep the kinetic chain open, usually using a weight machine.

B) Incorrect. Exercises that load the spine are classified as structural.

C) Incorrect. Exercises that keep either feet or hands at a fixed point are closed kinetic chain exercises; they close the kinetic chain.

D) Incorrect. Exercises that rely on a partner to stretch the limbs are PNF stretches (proprioceptive neuromuscular facilitation).

50. A) Incorrect. The chest is measured on men during the three-site skinfold measurement.

B) Incorrect. The abdomen is measured on men during the three-site skinfold measurement.

C) Correct. The thigh is measured during a woman's three-site skinfold measurement.

D) Incorrect. The subscapular region is measured during the seven-site skinfold measurement.

51.
A) Incorrect. The shoulders and upper back are not muscles that are assessed during the sit-and-reach test.

B) Incorrect. The shoulders are not assessed, but lower back flexibility is measured.

C) Incorrect. The quadriceps are not assessed, but lower back flexibility is measured.

D) Correct. Lower back and hamstring flexibility is assessed during the sit-and-reach test.

52.
A) Correct. This is the definition of eccentric muscle contraction.

B) Incorrect. This is the wrong type of muscle contraction.

C) Incorrect. This is the wrong type of muscle contraction.

D) Incorrect. This is the wrong type of muscle contraction.

53.
A) Incorrect. SMR is self-myofascial release.

B) Incorrect. Foam rolling is self-myofascial release.

C) Incorrect. Dynamic stretching includes active stretches that do not require assistance.

D) Correct. Proprioceptive neuromuscular facilitation does utilize a partner to aid in stretching muscles.

54.
A) Incorrect. This repetition range is too low for light loads.

B) Incorrect. This repetition range is too low for light loads.

C) Incorrect. This repetition range is too low for light loads.

D) Correct. For short rest periods and light loads, fifteen repetitions are appropriate.

55.
A) Incorrect. A warm-up should be less than moderate intensity.

B) Incorrect. A power training continuum workout is done at multiple intervals, not a warm-up.

C) **Correct.** The warm-up should prepare the body for stretching; it should be done at low to moderate intensity.

D) Incorrect. High intensity is appropriate for speed training or sprint training.

56.
A) **Correct.** Gender is a personal attribute and not an environmental factor.

B) Incorrect. Time is an environmental factor.

C) Incorrect. Weather is also an environmental factor that can be an exercise deterrent.

D) Incorrect. Social support is considered an environmental factor.

57.
A) Incorrect. The simplification of health insurance is one objective of HIPAA.

B) Correct. Protecting school records is an objective of FERPA, not HIPAA.

C) Incorrect. Protecting the privacy and security of healthcare information is one objective of HIPAA.

D) Incorrect. One objective of HIPAA is to streamline and minimize administrative costs.

58.
A) Incorrect. Supporting the wrists is not as safe as supporting the elbows.

B) Correct. Supporting the elbows is most effective for safety.

C) Incorrect. There is no need to support the neck for this exercise.

D) Incorrect. This is not a back-loaded exercise.

59.
A) Correct. Med ball chops and prisoner squats represent a full range of motion work at a higher intensity, with light or no weight, than a general cardio warm-up.

B) Incorrect. While arm circles could be considered a dynamic stretch, a deadlift is a structural core exercise using a moderate to heavy load.

C) Incorrect. While butt kickers could be considered a dynamic stretch, a hamstring static stretch is clearly a static stretch.

D) Incorrect. Both of these exercises are power moves and are too intense to be dynamic stretches.

60. **A)** **Correct.** This would be an effective cooldown protocol.

B) Incorrect. Collapsing on the floor in exhaustion risks the blood pooling and delayed onset muscle soreness.

C) Incorrect. Cooldowns should only involve body weight.

D) Incorrect. Static stretching or foam rolling should follow a session of lower intensity cardio.

61. **A)** **Correct.** Physician clearance should be required prior to beginning an exercise program for safety reasons.

B) Incorrect. The client may not know how serious the effects of that condition could be while exercising.

C) Incorrect. This is dangerous and the client could get hurt.

D) Incorrect. Unless the training manager is the client's primary physician, the manager should also not be training the client until the client has medical clearance to exercise.

62. A) Incorrect. Stabilization and strength training, not power training, focus on improving muscle endurance.

B) Incorrect. Strength training, not power training, focuses on building prime mover strength.

C) **Correct.** Power training focuses on muscle speed and force production.

D) Incorrect. Stabilization training, not power training, focuses on balance training.

63. A) Incorrect. Plyometrics is high intensity training that can be done in short bursts.

B) Incorrect. This lengthens muscles and doesn't usually elevate heart rate enough for aerobic endurance training.

C) Incorrect. Core training is a type of bodyweight resistance training, utilizing slow and controlled movement.

D) **Correct.** Circuit training can use various exercises in a continuous sequence with minimal rest causing an elevated heart rate for an extended period.

64. A) Incorrect. The readiness-to-change model focuses on cultivating a person's self-efficacy to facilitate behavior change.

B) Incorrect. The social cognitive theory model focuses on one person's observing a change in someone else to motivate his or her own decisions.

C) Incorrect. While the theory of planned behavior is closely related to the description, it does not focus on the whole environment, no matter how removed, as a factor in behavior change.

D) **Correct.** This is the correct descriptor for the socio-ecological model.

65. **A)** **Correct.** A straight leg deadlift is a more controlled hip hinge exercise than a kettlebell swing.

B) Incorrect. A box jump is an explosive hip flexion exercise.

C) Incorrect. A single-arm swing is a kettlebell swing using one arm, which is considered a progression.

D) Incorrect. A front raise is a shoulder exercise, not a hip and core exercise.

66. A) Incorrect. The triceps is a primary mover in a triceps extension.

B) **Correct.** The forearm is a primary mover for a wrist curl.

C) Incorrect. The shoulder is a primary mover for a lateral raise.

D) Incorrect. The biceps is a synergist muscle for the wrist curl.

67. **A)** **Correct.** A push press is an explosive, standing shoulder press, which is an advanced shoulder press.

B) Incorrect. While the primary movers are shoulders, the standing upright row is a pulling move, not a pushing move.

C)   Incorrect. The primary movers for a low row are the latissimus dorsi and the erector spinae.

D)   Incorrect. The primary mover for the push-up is the pectorals.

68. A)   Incorrect. This answer choice is only partially correct; ISSA is not accredited.

B)   Correct. NASM, ACE, and ACSM are the three top agencies in personal training certification.

C)   Incorrect. NCCA and ANSI are accreditation bureaus, and ISSA is not an accredited certifying body.

D)   Incorrect. This answer choice is only partially true. NSCA is not accredited and neither is it among the top agencies.

69. A)   Incorrect. A muscle knot causes muscle imbalance.

B)   Correct. Muscle imbalances create tightness around joints, leading to poor form and injury if not corrected.

C)   Incorrect. *Muscle explosion* is not a term.

D)   Incorrect. The structure of a muscle gives it its function for the body.

70. A)   Incorrect. The floor crunch lifts the head, neck, and shoulders, while the reverse crunch lifts the hip flexors and the pelvic floor; therefore the floor crunch is not the best regression for the reverse crunch.

B)   Incorrect. The floor crunch is performed in the semi-supine position, while the plank hold is performed in the prone position; therefore the floor crunch is not the best regression for the plank hold.

C)   Incorrect. The floor crunch lifts the head, neck, and shoulders, while the hip bridge lifts the glutes and the pelvic floor; therefore the floor crunch is not the best regression for the hip bridge.

D)   Correct. The floor crunch targets the same muscles and follows the same range of motion as the ball crunch; however the floor crunch allows for

more stabilization than the ball crunch. Thus it is an ideal regression for a client who is not ready for the controlled instability a stability ball provides.

71. A)   Incorrect. The palms are facing up on a supinated grip.

B)   Incorrect. In an alternating grip, one palm is up and the other is down.

C)   Incorrect. In a false grip, the palms are facing down.

D)   Correct. The palms are facing each other in a neutral grip.

72. A)   Incorrect. Nurses are part of the AHC.

B)   Incorrect. Psychologists are part of the AHC.

C)   Incorrect. Occupational therapists are part of the AHC.

D)   Correct. Psychics are not part of the AHC.

73. A)   Incorrect. The bench press is general and not very specific to the sport of basketball. It may be used during the very early stages of resistance training.

B)   Incorrect. The leg press is a stabilized movement that limits core involvement making it a poor choice for a basketball player.

C)   Correct. The plyometric squat jump is perfect for basketball players' peak performance because it is specific and will help to increase their jumping capabilities. The movement is used over and over in the course of a game of basketball.

D)   Incorrect. Rotator cuff exercises may be helpful in rehabilitation from shoulder injuries; however, it is not the most beneficial exercise for peak performance.

74. A)   Incorrect. The single leg windmill is a balance move and not a direct regression for the ball crunch.

B)   Incorrect. The full range of motion in a sit-up does not make this a direct regression.

C) **Correct.** Taking away the controlled instability of the ball makes the abdominal crunch the regression.

D) Incorrect. The primary mover for the rotation is the oblique muscles.

75. A) Incorrect. Short-distance sprints will help football players since the longest distance they run is one hundred yards.

B) **Correct.** Long-distance running does not follow the principle of specificity when it comes to football.

C) Incorrect. Power exercises that develop speed will improve football players' one-hundred-yard yard sprint time.

D) Incorrect. Muscular endurance exercises will help to benefit short-distance sprints.

76. A) Incorrect. A workout is the complete dynamic warm-up, training stimulus, cooldown, and stretching.

B) Incorrect. The load refers to the amount of weight being lifted in a set.

C) Incorrect. Overload is the principle that increases to training variables stimulates the muscle to adapt.

D) **Correct.** This is the definition of a set.

77. A) Incorrect. Progression is not the correct term.

B) **Correct.** There are typically rest periods between sets and exercises in a workout.

C) Incorrect. Range of motion is not the correct term.

D) Incorrect. Neither term is correct.

78. **A)** **Correct.** Detraining occurs more rapidly in the aspects of a cardiovascular training program.

B) Incorrect. There is a more gradual detraining in muscular strength and some is retained following a short period of exercise cessation.

C) Incorrect. Previously trained clients will retain some of their strength following cessation of a training program.

D) Incorrect. This will depend on the type of professional athlete, and any

muscular strength training will be retained slightly.

79. A) Incorrect. An increase in heart rate should be expected during the assessment.

B) **Correct.** If the client requests to stop, the personal trainer should terminate the test.

C) Incorrect. Perspiration may occur as the client is participating in physical activity.

D) Incorrect. The client may begin to experience fatigue during the assessment.

80. A) Incorrect. Push-and-pull routines use a variety of large muscle groups on opposing sides of the body, limiting the risk of muscular imbalances.

B) Incorrect. The bodyweight training program described includes exercises for both chest and back muscles, reducing the chance of one-dimensional training.

C) Incorrect. A trained yoga instructor will incorporate exercises to increase flexibility and utilize all the major muscle groups, reducing the risk of muscular imbalances.

D) **Correct.** Unilateral training programs have a high risk of causing muscular imbalances. A program focusing on the chest and anterior deltoids specifically can cause rounding of the shoulders and muscular imbalances of the upper body.

81. A) Incorrect. This should not be the main focus of a resistance training program for children and adolescents.

B) Incorrect. Specific and repetitive movements can cause overuse injuries even in children.

C) Incorrect. High-intensity exercise may be part of the sport they participate in, but technique and form are more important in their training programs.

D) **Correct.** Proper technique and form development should be the goal of child and adolescent resistance training programs.

82. A) Incorrect. Alternated grips are both underhanded and overhanded.

B) Incorrect. Supinated grips are underhanded.

C) Correct. A pronated grip is also known as an overhanded grip.

D) Incorrect. A clean grip requires wrist flexion: the palms are facing the ceiling and the fingers are supporting a barbell at the shoulders.

83. A) Incorrect. These are both progressions of the push-up due to fewer points of contact and an unstable surface.

B) Incorrect. These are both progressions due to the increased body weight lifted and a plyometric jump at the top.

C) Incorrect. These are both regressions that limit the weight lifted by the arms during a push-up.

D) Correct. The kneeling push-up is a regression whereas the push-up with feet elevated is a progression.

84. A) Incorrect. The strength test would not be the most important indicator of a client's ability to perform the activities of daily living.

B) Correct. The cardiorespiratory test will assess an individual's maximal oxygen consumption, which is an important physiological measurement.

C) Incorrect. A movement assessment would not be the most important indicator.

D) Incorrect. A static posture test will only determine how a client holds his or her body during stance.

85. A) Incorrect. The goal is specific in that the client wants to lose twenty-five pounds.

B) Incorrect. The goal is time-stamped in that the client wants to lose the weight in two months.

C) Correct. The goal is not realistic as this much weight loss is dangerous and unsustainable by healthy weight-loss methods.

D) Incorrect. The goal is measurable in that the client's weight is the measurement.

86. A) Incorrect. The client needs a physician's clearance since the assessment involves exercising.

B) Correct. The client should obtain a physician's clearance to participate in an exercise program that incorporates that joint.

C) Incorrect. This could lead to potential injury or muscular imbalances.

D) Incorrect. The client could be injured without supervision or advice, and should be instructed to ask a physician how to proceed.

87. A) Incorrect. PNF increases flexibility and can decrease strength and power performance, so it should be done at the end.

B) Incorrect. PNF should not be done during resistance training as it can have deleterious effects on strength and power.

C) Incorrect. PNF can cause decreased strength and power and can have a negative effect on running or other cardiovascular techniques.

D) Correct. PNF stretching should be saved for the end of the workout to improve flexibility.

88. A) Incorrect. Due to the lack of conditioning the opposite may be true.

B) Correct. Because novice clients lack conditioning, they may require more frequent and longer rest periods than advanced clients do.

C) Incorrect. Rest periods should be taken between exercises of the same muscle group and sets of the same exercise.

D) Incorrect. Rest periods should be taken between exercises of the same muscle group and sets of the same exercise.

89. A) Incorrect. Weight loads do not have any bearing on muscle isolation.

B) Incorrect. While breathing is a component of exercise technique, it is unrelated to muscle isolation.

C) Correct. The way the athlete grips barbells, machines, or free weights can help isolate muscle groups.

D) Incorrect. This is a way to use free weights, and can be combined with grips to work certain muscle groups.

90. A) Incorrect. An estimated maximum heart rate is used in the formula.

B) Correct. The formula is used to calculate the target heart rate for an activity.

C) Incorrect. The client's resting heart rate is used in the formula.

D) Incorrect. Heart rate recovery is determined using another method.

91. **A) Correct.** The 1RM is single repetition maximum to determine the client's maximal effort of strength for one repetition of an exercise.

B) Incorrect. The 1RM determines strength for a single exercise, not all exercises.

C) Incorrect. Target heart rate zone is determined by the Karvonen formula.

D) Incorrect. Although estimates can be made from the 1RM for submaximal efforts, the 1RM test is for a single repetition.

92. A) Incorrect. This test is administered prior to the program's implementation.

B) Correct. This test is administered periodically during a client's tenure with the trainer to determine progress.

C) Incorrect. This test is given to determine the overall success of an exercise program.

D) Incorrect. This information is given based on the midtest.

93. A) Incorrect. Increased lactate threshold is a long-term effect of anaerobic cardiovascular exercise.

B) Incorrect. Type II muscle fiber recruitment is a long-term effect of anaerobic cardiovascular exercise.

C) Correct. Both heart rate and respiration rate should increase during aerobic and anaerobic cardiovascular exercise.

D) Incorrect. Type I muscle fiber recruitment is a long-term effect of aerobic cardiovascular exercise.

94. A) Incorrect. This is not the correct representation of the CEC acronym.

B) Correct. CEC stands for *continuing education credit.*

C) Incorrect. The CEC acronym does not stand for *collective exercise collaboration.*

D) Incorrect. *Care education collective* is an incorrect representation of the acronym.

95. A) Incorrect. The second transition is a recovery period.

B) Incorrect. Sports-specific training occurs during the other three periods.

C) Incorrect. The athlete should still participate in physical activity in the second transition period.

D) Correct. The second transition period should involve active rest that includes non-specific recreational activities not related to the athlete's competition.

96. A) Incorrect. This is the definition of a pyramid set.

B) Incorrect. This is the definition of a multiple set program.

C) Correct. This is the definition of a superset.

D) Incorrect. This is the definition of circuit training.

97. A) Incorrect. Self-control can be considered discipline.

B) Incorrect. Willpower would also be considered discipline.

C) Incorrect. Self-love is a product of self-efficacy.

D) Correct. Self-efficacy is the ability to believe in oneself to achieve a goal.

98. A) **Correct.** Exercise specificity is extremely important for improvements in sports. The program should make sure to include sport-specific strength and conditioning.

B) Incorrect. Resistance training every day may lead to overtraining, depending on the sport.

C) Incorrect. This depends directly on the sport in which the athlete competes.

D) Incorrect. Though strength testing is important for many athletes, not all athletic improvement relies on it.

99. A) Incorrect. Injury is not an environmental factor.

B) Incorrect. Injury is not in the category of personal attributes.

C) **Correct.** Injury is categorized as a physical-activity factor.

D) Incorrect. Locus of control is a personal attribute.

100. A) Incorrect. Undulating periodization involves varying training protocols within a microcycle rather than for full microcycles.

B) Incorrect. This does not describe a type of periodization.

C) **Correct.** Steady progression of microcycles from endurance to power is a linear periodization.

D) Incorrect. Linear periodizations can be used for non-athlete clients.

101. A) Incorrect. This is for development of muscular strength.

B) Incorrect. This is for development of muscular endurance.

C) Incorrect. This will also develop muscular endurance.

D) **Correct.** The repetition range for muscular hypertrophy is eight to twelve repetitions.

102. A) **Correct.** Performing an exercise without compensation means the client is in the autonomous stage of learning.

B) Incorrect. This is the first stage of learning associated with extreme difficulty during the task.

C) Incorrect. This is not one of the stages of learning.

D) Incorrect. This is the second stage of learning associated with minor movement compensations, but the client is beginning to correct technique.

103. A) **Correct.** The forty-yard dash is used to measure maximal speed.

B) Incorrect. The three-hundred-yard shuttle is a cardiorespiratory test that measures anaerobic capacity.

C) Incorrect. The 1.5-mile run measures cardiovascular endurance.

D) Incorrect. The pro-shuttle test measures lateral speed and agility.

104. A) Incorrect. The client should be seated slightly upright.

B) Incorrect. Range of motion may be reduced by the client's physical changes; however, it does not need to be reduced dramatically.

C) Incorrect. Abdominal exercises should be encouraged for pregnant clients.

D) **Correct.** The client should be seated slightly upright.

105. A) **Correct.** Income is a personal attribute.

B) Incorrect. Income is not an environmental factor.

C) Incorrect. Income cannot be considered a physical-activity factor.

D) Incorrect. Income is not a core factor.

106. A) Incorrect. Resistance training effects are retained longer than cardiovascular gains after stopping an exercise program.

B) **Correct.** Cardiovascular gains are noticeably different only two weeks after training cessation.

C) Incorrect. Gender does not make a significant difference in detraining effects.

D) Incorrect. Gender does not make a significant difference in detraining effects.

107. A) **Correct.** Light to moderate cardiovascular exercise provides blood flow to the large muscle groups, making them more elastic and pliable for exercise.

B) Incorrect. Plyometrics are high intensity and could cause injury prior to dynamic stretching.

C) Incorrect. Agility exercises are high intensity and could cause injury prior to dynamic stretching.

D) Incorrect. Resistance training should be done after the warm-up and higher intensity exercises, such as plyometrics and agility training.

108. A) Incorrect. This is a matter of opinion and not one a personal trainer should decipher.

B) Incorrect. Intrinsic motivation typically has the longer-term goal of self-improvement and lifestyle change in mind.

C) Incorrect. Only body composition measurement, not a dress size, can truly indicate whether someone is obese.

D) **Correct.** External goals, based on outside motivators such as looking good in a wedding dress, are considered short-term goals and do not necessarily have long-term effects.

109. A) Incorrect. Zone training eventually increases in intensity as the client progresses.

B) Incorrect. The mode can change in zone training programs.

C) **Correct.** It provides exercise variance through different target heart rate zones and keeps the program interesting for the client.

D) Incorrect. It does not necessarily take less time than steady state and even starts by training the client in steady state.

110. A) Incorrect. Muscular power exercises may be too high intensity or high impact for senior citizens.

B) **Correct.** Exercises that make the activities of daily living easier are most beneficial for senior citizens and can help prevent injuries and falls.

C) Incorrect. Anaerobic endurance training may be too high intensity for senior citizens and may not be necessary to implement in their exercise program.

D) Incorrect. Arm strength may benefit seniors in some way, but due to difficulties with balance, a total body routine is more beneficial.

111. A) Incorrect. An internal locus of control is the belief that a person has control over his or her own life.

B) Incorrect. Intrinsic characterizes motivation.

C) **Correct.** Those with an external locus of control believe that outside forces control their lives.

D) Incorrect. This is not a locus of control descriptor.

112. A) Incorrect. According to the CDC, 20 percent is not the correct percentage.

B) Incorrect. The figure of 75 percent is not accurate, according to the CDC.

C) **Correct.** According to the CDC, 45 percent of adults in the US get the minimum recommended level of activity.

D) Incorrect. The figure of 90 percent is not accurate, according to the CDC.

113. A) Incorrect. Jumping rope is an advanced aerobic exercise.

B) Incorrect. Using the rowing machine is an advanced aerobic exercise.

C) **Correct.** Walking is the most fundamental form of aerobic exercise; it is ideal for people at any fitness level.

D) Incorrect. Running is an advanced form of aerobic exercise.

114.
A) Incorrect. While these are exercise adherence barriers, they are not considered the most difficult to overcome.

B) Incorrect. Self-efficacy is correct, but not accessibility.

C) Incorrect. Locus of control is correct, but intrinsic motivators is not.

D) Correct. Self-efficacy and locus of control are considered the most difficult exercise adherence barriers to overcome.

115.
A) Incorrect. Steady-state cardiovascular training does little to improve lactate threshold.

B) Incorrect. Maximal strength resistance training helps improve muscular strength.

C) Incorrect. Muscular power training helps develop speed but not lactate threshold.

D) Correct. Sprint interval training will help to improve lactate threshold.

116.
A) Incorrect. According to the CDC, twenty-nine percent of adults in the US are overweight.

B) Incorrect. Among adults in the US, six percent are morbidly obese, according to the CDC.

C) Incorrect. Only thirty-one percent of adults in the US are a healthy weight.

D) Correct. Thirty-four percent of adults in the US are obese, according to the CDC.

117.
A) Incorrect. Though some fitness websites may list emergency action plans, an appropriate resource with the governing rules and regulations is more credible.

B) Incorrect. Fitness professionals may have different plans set in place for one facility or place of work, and the information will vary for every individual.

C) Correct. The US Department of Labor website lists the minimum requirements for an employer's facility emergency action plan. Various factors will increase the regulations each employer will follow, but the employer's action plan must at least meet the minimum requirements.

D) Incorrect. Local business action plans will vary based on the company size and number of employees. Additionally, these companies may not be following the government rules and regulations and could be subject to litigation themselves. It is best to go straight to the source.

118.
A) Incorrect. Three weeks is not accurate.

B) Incorrect. Two months is not the correct answer.

C) Correct. Among individuals adhering to a fitness program, 50 percent drop the program after six months.

D) Incorrect. Eight months is not the correct response.

119.
A) Incorrect. Age is a personal attribute.

B) Correct. Accessibility is an environmental factor.

C) Incorrect. Time is a personal attribute.

D) Incorrect. Fitness level is a personal attribute.

120. A) Correct. Cueing involves the use of specific movements and words as outlined in this definition.

B) Incorrect. This definition does not apply to exercise.

C) Incorrect. Phrasing does not include using these actions.

D) Incorrect. This is not the definition of sign language.

121.
A) Incorrect. Information stored on a trainer's phone is not accessible to other employees and could be lost if the phone is damaged.

B) Incorrect. Keeping the information on an email list does not allow for quick access to the information in emergency situations.

C) Incorrect. Work computers often have multiple users, and the emergency contact information could be lost among the files or accessed by another user, compromising client privacy.

D) Correct. Keeping files alphabetized in a filing cabinet allows for easy access in case of an emergency, and locking the cabinet ensures the files stay secure.

122. A) Incorrect. In the precontemplation phase, the participant hasn't even thought of change.

B) Incorrect. In the maintenance phase, the participant has already acted and is continuing this action successfully, being mindful of relapses.

C) Correct. This is the correct descriptor of the action phase.

D) Incorrect. In the preparation phase, the participant is planning to act within a month.

123. A) Incorrect. Rock climbing does not necessarily increase the risk of medial knee injuries in female athletes.

B) Correct. Jumping increases the risk of medial knee injuries in female athletes with increased Q-angles.

C) Incorrect. Ice hockey does not necessarily increase the risk of medial knee injuries in female athletes.

D) Incorrect. Snowboarding does not necessarily increase the risk of medial knee injuries in female athletes.

124. A) Incorrect. It is possible to use college courses to earn CEC requirements.

B) Incorrect. Industry specialization certifications can be used to obtain CEC points.

C) Correct. Contributing to a scholarly article is an acceptable way to earn CECs, but contributing to a blog is not; blogs are not considered scholarly.

D) Incorrect. It is possible to apply accredited programs' learning modules to obtain CEC points.

125. A) Incorrect. *Mode of specialty* is a term used in the military and does not pertain to personal trainers.

B) Incorrect. Physical location does not influence the advice given.

C) Correct. Health professionals have limitations based on their certifications or licensure.

D) Incorrect. This term does not describe a personal trainer's certified or licensed specialty.

126. A) Incorrect. Kinesthetic feedback is not an actual type of feedback.

B) Incorrect. Positive reinforcement is not necessarily specific.

C) Correct. This is the correct description of targeted praise.

D) Incorrect. The description is not limited to just non-verbal communication.

127. A) Incorrect. Liability insurance covers defamation.

B) Incorrect. Liability insurance covers invasion of privacy.

C) Incorrect. Neither liability nor miscellaneous insurance covers wrongful termination.

D) Correct. Miscellaneous personal trainer's insurance covers bodily injury.

128. A) Correct. This is the correct descriptor of the preparation phase.

B) Incorrect. In the contemplation phase, the participant has decided not to be stuck in the same unhealthy rut.

C) Incorrect. In the action phase, the participant has reached the goal and will continue to change as part of his or her lifestyle.

D) Incorrect. Initiation does not occur during termination.

129. A) Incorrect. Only *rapport* is correct.

B) Incorrect. Only *empathy* is correct.

C) Incorrect. Only *rapport* and *assessment* are correct.

D) Correct. The READ acronym represents *rapport, empathy, assessment,* and *development.*

130. A) Incorrect. Hormones are what an organ secretes, but they are not the organ itself.

B) Incorrect. The brain contains glands, but it is not a gland itself.

C) Incorrect. This is a hormone that is secreted by a gland.

D) Correct. This is the definition of a gland.

131. A) Incorrect. This is not a common side effect of anabolic steroid abuse.

B) Incorrect. This is not a common side effect of anabolic steroid abuse.

C) Correct. Anabolic steroid abuse can damage the liver.

D) Incorrect. This is not a common side effect of anabolic steroid abuse.

132. A) Correct. Fire alarms are typically linked directly to emergency authorities, so the response will be fast.

B) Incorrect. The appropriate personnel may not hear a shout for help.

C) Incorrect. Calling a friend creates an additional step in alerting emergency personnel and will increase the response time.

D) Incorrect. Email is not always readily available and will increase the response time.

133. A) Correct. This plyometric exercise is specific to running, and the first transition period should incorporate higher intensity exercises to start building to peak performance during the competitive period.

B) Incorrect. A standard wall sit is not very specific and should be incorporated in the beginning of the preparatory period for beginners.

C) Incorrect. Barbell bench press is a basic strength training exercise that is most beneficial at the beginning of the training program.

D) Incorrect. The triceps kickback is not very specific to triathletes, especially during the first transition period.

134. A) Incorrect. Injuries involving severe bleeding require cleaning the wound, applying a sterile dressing, and possibly seeking medical assistance.

B) Correct. RICE stands for **R**est, **I**ce, **C**ompression, and **E**levation. This acronym should be followed in caring for sprains, strains, and contusions.

C) Incorrect. Cardiopulmonary issues may be serious and require emergency responders.

D) Incorrect. Chest pain can indicate serious problems such as a heart attack and may require emergency responders.

135. A) Incorrect. *Exercise selection* is not a real term.

B) Incorrect. This is not the correct description of motivation.

C) Correct. Exercise adherence involves a voluntary commitment to an exercise program.

D) Incorrect. *Exercise commitment* is not an actual term, just a rewording of the description.

136. A) **Correct.** The trainer should increase the difficulty of the exercise by implementing a progression of the same exercise.

B) Incorrect. A regression would have the opposite effect, decreasing the chances of reaching fitness goals.

C) Incorrect. Stopping exercise after mastering a particular technique will not help the client reach their goals. New goals should be set and achieved.

D) Incorrect. Although a totally new workout may give the client some variety, it will be more difficult to see training progress than simply implementing a progression of the same exercise.

137. A) Incorrect. This is glucose.

B) Incorrect. This is the coenzyme that goes through the Krebs cycle.

C) Incorrect. This is used for immediate synthesis of ATP in the muscles within the first seconds of exercise.

D) Correct. This is the definition of glycogen.

138. A) Incorrect. Income does not fall into the environmental factor category.

B) Correct. Income is a personal attribute.

C) Incorrect. Self-efficacy is not a category; it is a personal attribute.

D) Incorrect. Income is not among the physical-activity factors.

139. A) Incorrect. This is not an example of a first-class lever.

B) Incorrect. The calf raise utilizes a type of lever.

C) Correct. The calf raise is an example of a second-class lever.

D) Incorrect. This is not an example of a third-class lever.

140. A) Incorrect. Clients should be encouraged to exercise at a comfortable pace based on their assessments.

B) Incorrect. Not all clients will enjoy more difficult workouts; this is highly variable.

C) Incorrect. The best way to ensure the client is getting good value is to make sure the client is exercising in a healthy and effective manner and not always doing a high-intensity workout.

D) Correct. Monitoring intensity is a means of reducing risks associated with exercise.

141. A) Incorrect. Movement assessments do not test maximal force.

B) Incorrect. Movement assessments do not test core strength.

C) Incorrect. Movement assessments do not test agility and speed.

D) Correct. Movement assessments are used to test dynamic posture.

142. A) Incorrect. The belief step in planning cannot aid the trainer this way.

B) Incorrect. The vision step does not help the trainer determine how close a client is to meeting his or her goals.

C) Correct. The learning step in planning does help the trainer determine how close a client is to meeting his or her goals.

D) Incorrect. The persistence step in planning would not be used to determine this.

143. A) Incorrect. Using password protection is a proper security procedure.

B) Incorrect. Anti-virus protection is among the proper security procedures.

C) Correct. Leaving electronic devices accessible to employees will not provide the proper security to protect confidential information.

D) Incorrect. Installing software for malware detection is a proper security procedure.

144. **A) Correct.** It is good practice to be well protected against injury, defamation and negligence.

B) Incorrect. This is not necessary for a personal trainer unless the trainer wants to teach group fitness.

C) Incorrect. A trainer at a gym should not need to buy additional equipment.

D) Incorrect. A trainer does not need a social media account.

145. A) Incorrect. A personal trainer should not participate in gossip.

B) Correct. Personal trainers obtain sensitive information from their clients.

C) Incorrect. Personal trainers should not find clients' sensitive personal information humorous.

D) Incorrect. While personal trainers do receive basic information, much of it is better classified as sensitive.

146. A) Incorrect. This is a supinated grip.

B) Correct. The thumb wraps around the same side as the fingers.

C) Incorrect. This is a hook grip.

D) Incorrect. This is the same as a supinated grip.

147. A) Incorrect. Free weights use gravity and the body's concentric and isometric force.

B) Incorrect. Hydraulic machines use compressed air or water resistance.

C) Incorrect. Suspension trainers use bodyweight, gravity, and leverage.

D) Correct. Cam machines use a combination of body movement, gravity, and friction to work the body.

148. A) Incorrect. A sedentary lifestyle is a potential risk factor.

B) Incorrect. High blood pressure is a risk factor that may require the client to get medical clearance.

C) Correct. A low resting heart rate is NOT a risk factor that could require medical clearance.

D) Incorrect. Obesity is a risk factor, and new clients with this condition may require medical clearance.

149. A) Incorrect. Fitness professionals will benefit more from a BLS course that also includes AED and first aid.

B) Incorrect. Fitness professionals will benefit more from a BLS course that also includes first aid and CPR.

C) Correct. BLS classes for fitness professionals should include first aid, CPR, and AED training.

D) Incorrect. Evaluating cardiac arrhythmias is beyond the scope of most certified personal training settings.

150. A) Incorrect. Exercise advice is within a personal trainer's scope of practice.

B) Incorrect. A personal trainer's scope of practice includes providing advice on stretching.

C) Incorrect. Providing advice on general health matters is within a personal trainer's scope of practice.

D) Correct. Providing nutrition advice does not fall within a personal trainer's scope of practice unless the trainer has additional certification in nutrition.

TWO: Practice Test Two

READ THE QUESTION, AND THEN CHOOSE THE MOST CORRECT ANSWER.

1. Which of the following tests requires a spotter?

   A) balance error scoring system

   B) single-leg squat

   C) star excursion balance test

   D) overhead squat

2. Which of the answer choices below does NOT describe a function of the bones?

   A) They store necessary minerals.

   B) They protect internal organs.

   C) They synthesize blood cells.

   D) They produce force for movement.

3. Center of gravity refers to

   A) the area directly under the body, including where the body contacts the ground.

   B) the area where the least amount of body weight is located.

   C) an imaginary point on the body in which body weight is completely and evenly distributed in relation to the ground.

   D) the direct center point between a person's feet.

4. What muscular action occurs at the forearm when the palm is rotated to face upward?

   A) pronation

   B) supination

   C) abduction

   D) flexion

5. Which of the following refers to muscles that assist the muscular agonists when performing a movement?

   A) antagonists

   B) stabilizers

   C) neutralizers

   D) synergists

6. Which of the following measurements can be used to identify individuals who are at a greater risk of diseases, such as coronary heart disease and type two diabetes?

   A) waist-to-hip ratio

   B) the Rockport walk test

   C) BMI

   D) balance error scoring system

7. Which of the following is NOT a cardiorespiratory assessment?

   A) the *t*-test
   B) 1.5-mile run test
   C) three-minute step test
   D) Rockport walk test

8. According to the force-velocity curve, an increase in force provides improvement to

   A) muscular strength.
   B) muscular endurance.
   C) muscular power.
   D) muscular speed.

9. Which of these tests is used to measure a client's stretch-shortening cycle effort?

   A) long jump
   B) reactive strength index
   C) forty-yard dash
   D) hexagon

10. Free weights include all the following EXCEPT:

    A) kettlebells
    B) dumbbells
    C) sandbags
    D) treadmills

11. Which of the following is NOT a macronutrient?

    A) carbohydrate
    B) protein
    C) fat
    D) vitamin

12. Delayed onset muscle soreness (DOMS) is caused by

    A) lactic acid buildup in the muscles.
    B) static stretching.
    C) micro-tears in the muscle fibers.
    D) a sedentary lifestyle.

13. What question should a trainer continue asking to help the client uncover his or her true, intrinsic motivator?

    A) How?
    B) Really?
    C) Why?
    D) And?

14. Deficiency of what vitamin can lead to poor bone density?

    A) vitamin D
    B) vitamin A
    C) vitamin C
    D) vitamin K

15. What information is the health history questionnaire used to collect?

    A) previous exercise experience
    B) general health information
    C) lifestyle information
    D) occupational information

16. A machine leg extension is an example of what type of movement?

    A) closed kinetic chain movement
    B) core exercise
    C) open kinetic chain movement
    D) transverse movement

17. The neuroendocrine response to exercise is elicited by

A) working smaller muscle groups, like the biceps or triceps.

B) performing single joint exercises, like wrist curls.

C) performing light cardiovascular exercise, such as walking.

D) performing large muscle group exercises, like the deadlift.

18. Which blood pressure measurements would be a risk factor for developing cardiovascular disease?

A) 120/80

B) 115/75

C) 130/70

D) 140/90

19. Which two actions do the quadriceps muscles perform?

A) knee flexion and hip flexion

B) knee extension and hip flexion

C) knee flexion and hip extension

D) knee extension and hip extension

20. When designing an athlete's cardiovascular training program, it is important to keep in mind

A) athletes should all do steady-state cardio.

B) athletes should all do interval training.

C) the work-to-rest ratio of their sport.

D) cardio is not as important as resistance training in sports.

21. Which term below best refers to poor bone mineral density due to the loss or lack of production of calcium content and bone cells, which leads to bone brittleness?

A) rheumatoid arthritis

B) arthritis

C) osteoporosis

D) postural deviation

22. Which athlete will benefit from fast-twitch muscle fibers the most?

A) marathoners

B) 1500-meter swimmers

C) Olympic sprinters

D) cross-country cyclists

23. Which exercise may require a spotter?

A) barbell deadlift

B) medicine ball slam

C) back-loaded squat

D) walking lunges

24. When creating an exercise program, which form will most accurately help the personal trainer identify the client's goals?

A) medical clearance

B) lifestyle questionnaire

C) body composition test

D) health history

25. Which connect chain checkpoint compensation reveals lower crossed syndrome?

A) shoulders

B) foot and ankle

C) head and cervical spine

D) lumbo/pelvic/hip complex

26. Which type of athletes are at risk for iron-deficiency anemia?

   A) both strength and endurance athletes

   B) male athletes

   C) strength athletes, female athletes, and vegetarians

   D) endurance athletes, female athletes, and vegetarians

27. Box jumps, tuck jumps, and backward skips are examples of what type of training?

   A) agility

   B) plyometrics

   C) cardiorespiratory

   D) circuit

28. A typical mesocycle may last

   A) six to twelve weeks.

   B) one week.

   C) an entire year.

   D) nearly two years.

29. Which of the following is NOT a function of protein in the body?

   A) It makes up muscle fibers.

   B) It composes enzymes that catalyze chemical reactions.

   C) It makes up receptors in cell membranes that transmit hormonal messages to cells.

   D) It is the major structural component of cell membranes.

30. Which compensations should the personal trainer look for at the foot and ankle while observing the client from the anterior view?

   A) not adducted or abducted

   B) not flattened or externally rotated

   C) not anteriorly or posteriorly rotated

   D) neither tilted nor rotated

31. Which cardiorespiratory fitness assessment would most accurately measure anaerobic capacity?

   A) 300-yard shuttle

   B) twelve-minute run

   C) three-minute step test

   D) 1.5-mile run

32. How soon after starting a resistance training program can neuromuscular benefits be seen?

   A) after the first session

   B) after several weeks

   C) after four weeks

   D) after six weeks

33. Which cycle is the shortest of a periodization program?

   A) the mesocycle

   B) the macrocycle

   C) the microcycle

   D) the preparatory period

34. What are disordered heart rhythms called?

   A) arrhythmias

   B) amenorrhea

   C) hypertension

   D) atherosclerosis

35. Which description best represents static posture?

  A) how an individual physically moves

  B) how an individual maintains alignment while moving

  C) how individuals present themselves in stance

  D) posture during exercise

36. Which of the following describes the type of validity that represents the extent to which test scores are related to those of other accepted tests that measure the same ability?

  A) content validity

  B) criterion-referenced validity

  C) face validity

  D) concurrent validity

37. The belief step in planning is intended to help the client manage _____ and _____.

  A) fear, pride

  B) relapse, recovery phase

  C) relapse, self-doubt

  D) fear, self-doubt

38. Which test is the most effective for assessing speed, agility, and quickness?

  A) Rockport walk test

  B) push-up test

  C) hexagon test

  D) twelve-minute run test

39. Which lifestyle choice is considered the leading cause of preventable death according to the Centers for Disease Control and Prevention (CDC)?

  A) stress level

  B) alcohol consumption

  C) exercise practices

  D) smoking

40. All of the following tests are used to measure speed, agility, and quickness EXCEPT

  A) the 300-yard shuttle test.

  B) the LEFT.

  C) the pro-agility test.

  D) the *t*-test.

41. Which of the following is NOT checked on the body during a static assessment?

  A) optimal alignment

  B) muscle symmetry

  C) overhead squat posturing

  D) balanced muscle tone

42. What is the common PNF stretching sequence?

  A) stretch-release

  B) hold-relax

  C) relax-breathe

  D) contract-contract

43. What is the most appropriate assessment for a prenatal client?

  A) bench press

  B) single-leg squat

  C) gait

  D) forty-yard dash

44. What are the two most common anatomical sites to measure the heart rate?

  A) brachial and radial

  B) carotid and brachial

  C) radial and femoral

  D) carotid and radial

45. What is/are the first source(s) of energy during a sprint?

A) muscle glycogen

B) intramuscular triglycerides

C) phosphocreatine and ATP

D) liver glycogen

46. Which test would best measure a youth client's speed, agility, and quickness?

A) pro-agility test

B) barbell squat test

C) single-leg squat assessment

D) push-up test

47. Which statement below does NOT describe the use of the social support behavioral modification technique?

A) doing a positive behavior to avoid a negative consequence of a negative behavior

B) enlist a friend to be a workout buddy

C) create a social media group for healthy recipe swapping

D) have a friend or a family member on-call if feeling vulnerable

48. Which of the following muscles is NOT part of the movement system of the core?

A) transversus abdominis

B) hip flexors

C) erector spinae

D) abductor complex

49. Which of the following assessments does NOT measure body fat percentage?

A) dual-energy x-ray absorptiometry (DEXA)

B) body mass index (BMI)

C) near-infrared interactance

D) air displacement plethysmography (BOD POD)

50. Which of the following types of validity refers to a test that appears to measure what it is intended to measure?

A) concurrent validity

B) discriminant validity

C) content validity

D) face validity

51. The BMI might NOT be an accurate indicator of a healthy weight

A) when the individual is tall.

B) when the individual is short.

C) if the individual is a strength trainer.

D) if the individual is sedentary.

52. Which of the following body groups allows the personal trainer to systematically view the body in an organized manner?

A) joint mobility chains

B) skeletal categorizations

C) arthrokinematic checkpoints

D) kinetic chain checkpoints

53. Excessive lateral curvature of the spine is referred to as

A) scoliosis.

B) lordosi.

C) osteoporosis.

D) kyphosis.

54. Which of the following will be discussed during the lifestyle questionnaire?

A) readiness for activity

B) medical problems

C) medications used

D) stressors

55. What are the regions that are measured during the three-site skinfold assessment with a female client?

A) chest, biceps, thigh

B) triceps, suprailium, thigh

C) subscapular, thigh, suprailium

D) biceps, thigh, suprailium

56. Because of their deadline, which type of goals keep the client motivated?

A) time-bound

B) challenging

C) proximal

D) realistic

57. Which of the following is NOT within a certified fitness professional's scope of practice?

A) fitness assessment

B) program design

C) massage therapy

D) goal-setting

58. The dynamic warm-up should implement exercises that

A) prepare all of the muscles that will be trained during the workout.

B) improve flexibility.

C) are basic and not specific.

D) increase muscular power.

59. Which assessment would be most appropriate for a sixty-five-year-old client who wants to lower his or her blood pressure?

A) bench press test

B) hexagon test

C) Rockport walk test

D) three-hundred-yard shuttle test

60. Which test helps determine an individual's ability to change direction and stabilize the body at high speeds?

A) hexagon test

B) t-test

C) pro-agility test

D) vertical jump test

61. It is important to focus on form and _____ before loading the body with heavy weight loads.

A) body control

B) breathing

C) flexibility

D) positive outlook

62. What is the starting position for a power drop?

A) supine

B) sitting

C) semi-supine

D) prone

63. During an overhead squat assessment, which of the following compensations CANNOT be viewed posteriorly?

A) lateral movement of the feet

B) excessive foot pronation

C) heels lift from the floor

D) asymmetrical weight shift in the hips

64. Successful people do not give up, no matter how hard they must work or how many times they make mistakes; this is _____.

A) love

B) fear

C) locus of control

D) persistence

65. Strength training should follow a progressive plan with three tiers, which are _____, _____, and _____.

A) power, muscle, matter

B) strength, power, hard

C) stabilization, strength, power

D) stabilization, body, strength

66. A barbell deadlift or a rear loaded squat can be considered _____ exercises.

A) structural

B) power

C) agility

D) assistance

67. Which of the following is NOT true of the drawing-in maneuver?

A) It aids in core activation.

B) It maintains neutral posturing.

C) It is used for all core exercises.

D) It stretches the hip flexors.

68. The body's ability to move in one direction as quickly as possible is

A) agility.

B) force.

C) speed.

D) power.

69. Which of the following does the overhead squat test NOT assess?

A) neuromuscular efficiency

B) functional strength

C) unilateral balance

D) dynamic flexibility

70. Which type of exercises typically activates smaller muscle groups and is used for rehabilitative purposes?

A) core exercises

B) open kinetic chain exercises

C) PNF stretching

D) assistance exercises

71. How might the trainer progress an already difficult exercise, such as a single-leg squat?

A) There is no further progression.

B) Add a box to sit down on.

C) Add weight with a vest or dumbbells.

D) Pick a new exercise to perform.

72. What is the connection and cohesive function of all three body systems—the nervous system, the muscular system, and the skeletal system?

A) neuromuscular efficiency

B) progressive system

C) kinetic chain

D) postural balance

73. Which of the following is NOT a relative contraindication?

A) uncontrollable metabolic disease

B) symptomatic heart failure

C) musculoskeletal disorder

D) history of heart illness

74. In which situation would a personal trainer need to immediately refer a client to a medical professional?

A) a client complains of lower back pain

B) a client complains of anterior knee pain

C) a client has had recent complications with cardiac disease

D) a client does not feel well

75. Which type of stretching helps to elicit an elongation of the muscle fibers and improved flexibility?

A) dynamic stretching

B) static stretching

C) self-myofascial release

D) dynamic warm-up

76. High-volume and low-load muscular endurance training can cause fatigue and should be saved for the

A) in-season.

B) off-season.

C) competitive period.

D) second transition period.

77. When should static stretching be performed in a workout?

A) prior to exercise

B) before the plyometrics

C) before the cardiovascular exercise

D) at the end of the workout

78. What is a repetition?

A) The performance of an exercise multiple times through its full range of motion.

B) The amount of weight used for an exercise.

C) The number of exercises used in a workout.

D) The performance of an exercise through its full range of motion one time.

79. A dynamic warm-up for a field hockey player should include these three things:

A) static stretching, dynamic stretching, and cardiovascular exercise

B) dynamic stretching, single-muscle group exercises, and plyometrics

C) five minutes of aerobic exercise, dynamic stretching, and specific movement patterns of the workout

D) dynamic stretching, PNF stretching, and foam rolling

80. A circuit-training program involving a careful selection of varying muscle groups to minimize rest periods is called

A) horizontal loading.

B) single set.

C) interval training.

D) vertical loading.

81. For a training program to follow the principle of overload it needs to

A) maintain training loads throughout the program.

B) gradually increase training loads throughout the program.

C) decrease training loads throughout the program.

D) rapidly increase training loads throughout the program.

82. Why should power exercises be performed prior to muscular endurance exercises?

    A) to promote flexibility

    B) power exercises are lower intensity and should be performed first

    C) muscular endurance exercises are higher intensity and should be performed last

    D) power exercises require high levels of technique, and muscular endurance exercises can cause fatigue and decreased performance quality

83. The RPE scale is a subjective scale measuring

    A) how much exercise the client is performing.

    B) what mode of exercise the client is performing.

    C) how difficult the client feels the exercise is.

    D) the client's opinion of the workout for the day.

84. How many points of contact should a client have when lying in a semi-supine position?

    A) 7

    B) 3

    C) 4

    D) 5

85. In the relapse prevention and recovery plan techniques of behavior change, the ABC model of behavior helps to identify _____ for unwanted or desired activities.

    A) triggers

    B) obsessions

    C) irritants

    D) successes

86. As training volume decreases, load

    A) increases.

    B) decreases.

    C) stays the same.

    D) does not change because the two variables are not associated.

87. What are the two important types of hormones associated with exercise?

    A) anabolic and testosterone

    B) anabolic and IGF

    C) anabolic and epinephrine

    D) anabolic and catabolic

88. What is a training plateau?

    A) a decrease in the difficulty of an exercise due to physical limitation

    B) a high point in the training program where a goal is achieved

    C) an increase in exercise difficulty designed to overload the muscles

    D) a point in a client's training program associated with no positive gains from exercise

89. _____ is the body's ability to react to a cue that propels a change in direction.

    A) Agility

    B) Quickness

    C) Readiness

    D) Stabilization

90. A network of licensed, certified, or registered professionals who provide healthcare resources to the general population is called what?

    A) allied healthcare continuum

    B) training continuum

    C) health professionals

    D) health maintenance professionals

91. Plyometric exercises are also referred to as
    A) strength training.
    B) force training.
    C) quickness training.
    D) power training.

92. What muscles are targeted in a lateral pulldown?
    A) transversus abdominis
    B) latissimus dorsi
    C) anterior deltoids
    D) quadriceps

93. Which of the following is NOT an example of relapse prevention and recovery plans?
    A) use the ABC model of behavior to identify triggers
    B) plan a weekly menu and shopping list to eliminate the need for a fast food meal
    C) do NOT focus on fault
    D) create a contingency plan for social outings

94. Program design for weight management should include
    A) resistance training and nutrition.
    B) cardiovascular training and nutrition.
    C) nutrition only.
    D) warm-up, resistance training, cardiovascular training, nutrition, cooldown, and recovery methods.

95. A macrocycle includes
    A) only the in-season program.
    B) the entirety of a training periodization.
    C) only off-season training.
    D) only the preparatory period of training.

96. Which of the following is NOT an example of the self-monitoring behavior modification technique?
    A) diet journaling
    B) activity tracking
    C) rewarding completion of a goal
    D) incorporating weekly weigh-ins

97. Verbal communication comprises only _____ of how we express ourselves.
    A) 7 percent
    B) 10 percent
    C) 55 percent
    D) 38 percent

98. Periodization programs should strive to have the athlete peak
    A) throughout the entirety of the program.
    B) at the beginning of the program.
    C) just prior to competition or major events such as tryouts.
    D) Peak performance should not be reached because it is potentially harmful to the client.

99. In which phases of the readiness-to-change model will clients need to use behavior modification tools to keep them on track?
    A) maintenance and termination phases
    B) action and precontemplation phases
    C) action and maintenance phases
    D) contemplation and preparation phases

100. Since children have difficulty regulating their body temperature, it is important to make sure

A) they are exercising outdoors.

B) they exercise only when it is cold out.

C) they are hydrating properly.

D) they are exercising indoors.

101. Obese clients may need to avoid which exercises due to excessive stress placed on the joints?

A) muscular power exercises, such as Olympic lifts and plyometrics

B) muscular endurance exercises with low loads and high volume

C) muscular strength exercises with heavy loads and low volumes

D) muscular hypertrophy exercises because they will increase the client's body weight, further adding to the stress

102. During a dynamic warm-up, the dynamic movements should include about

A) fifteen repetitions per side of each exercise.

B) one or two repetitions per side of each exercise.

C) ten to twenty repetitions per side of each exercise.

D) five repetitions per side of each exercise.

103. What type of aerobic exercise should be included in programs focused on general health benefits?

A) running only

B) cycling and swimming only

C) all modes are beneficial

D) general health benefits do not require aerobic exercise

104. How might the trainer regress a bodyweight squat exercise?

A) add weights with a vest or dumbbells

B) add a jump to the top of the range of motion

C) perform a bodyweight Romanian deadlift

D) perform a wall sit or wall slide exercise

105. When performing supersets, which combination of exercises would be most appropriate?

A) lunges and step-ups

B) push and push

C) pull and push

D) push-ups and bench press

106. A program containing muscular strength, muscular endurance, and muscular hypertrophy within a single microcycle is considered what?

A) linear periodization

B) undulating periodization

C) exercise regression

D) dangerous

107. Sandbags, resistance tubes, and stability balls are what types of equipment?

A) transitional

B) cardio

C) functional

D) controlled

108. Program design for clients with chronic back pain should emphasize

A) upper body resistance training.

B) core muscle endurance and flexibility training.

C) lower body resistance training.

D) avoiding the low back entirely.

109. What is the first step in building professional client relationships?

   A) giving a good assessment

   B) building rapport

   C) using positive body language

   D) giving a high five and a smile

110. Periods in a periodization follow this order:

   A) preparatory period, competitive period, first transition period, second transition period

   B) macrocycle, microcycle, mesocycle

   C) competitive period, first transition period, second transition period, preparatory period

   D) preparatory period, first transition period, competitive period, second transition period

111. To reduce the risk of liability in a potential lawsuit, fitness professionals should require that new clients complete which of the following?

   A) medical history forms, a liability waiver, informed consent to exercise, and a PAR-Q

   B) medical history forms, favorite hobbies, a bloodwork form, and a PAR-Q

   C) medical history forms, a liability waiver, informed consent, and a bloodwork form

   D) medical history forms, a liability waiver, a PAR-Q, and a fitness assessment

112. Which of the following is NOT a positive body language indicator?

   A) nodding slowly or quickly

   B) leaning forward

   C) wringing hands

   D) firm handshake

113. Why might plyometrics not be advisable for individuals who are overweight or obese?

   A) They develop muscular power.

   B) They are not fun.

   C) They are too easy.

   D) They place excessive force on the joints.

114. Non-verbal communication generally consists of

   A) vocal tone and words.

   B) body language and singing skills.

   C) vocal tone and body language.

   D) words and body language.

115. Low self-efficacy and external locus of control dominate people in the _____ phase; they believe their situations are hopeless and they would rather ignore them.

   A) preparation

   B) precontemplation

   C) action

   D) termination

116. Which of the following is NOT a negative body language indicator?

   A) finger tapping

   B) tall posture

   C) shifting eyes

   D) arms crossed

117. The last part of a warm-up should consist of what type of stretching?

   A) static stretching

   B) PNF stretching

   C) dynamic stretching

   D) SMR stretching

118. In general, the code of ethics for personal trainers applies to all the following areas, EXCEPT which one?

A) professionalism

B) confidentiality

C) friendship

D) business practices

119. Which of the following does NOT refer to body language?

A) facial expressions

B) vocal quality

C) words spoken

D) posture

120. When meeting with a client, the trainer should exude

A) cockiness, enthusiasm, and joy.

B) confidence, enthusiasm, and professionalism.

C) confidence, assertiveness, and likeability.

D) pride, love, and goodness.

121. With resistance training, the intensity increases as the

A) weight decreases.

B) volume increases.

C) weight increases.

D) repetitions increase.

122. A professional trainer would wear which of the following?

A) khaki pants or jeans

B) tasteful athletic attire

C) revealing athletic attire

D) strong cologne or perfume

123. The practice of active listening means _____ and _____ _____ are occurring while working with a client.

A) verbal, non-verbal communication

B) positive, negative body language

C) empathy, rapport building

D) core, structural exercises

124. When using active listening, a trainer should do what after the client has finished his statement or question?

A) Give him a high five and a smile.

B) Give him a hug.

C) Walk away nodding.

D) Repeat key elements of the client's statement.

125. A personal training certification typically needs to be renewed every _____ years.

A) one

B) four

C) six

D) two

126. Minimizing opportunities that trigger unwanted behavior in order to maximize desired behavior is called

A) stimulus control.

B) socio-ecological theory.

C) self-monitoring.

D) locus of control.

127. The technique of setting reasonable and attainable goals to inhibit unsuccessful results is an example of

A) self-monitoring.

B) cognitive coping.

C) reward.

D) negative reinforcement.

128. While it is important for trainers to be positive, it is also important for them to be _____.

A) pragmatic
B) right
C) negative
D) social

129. Using one day of the week to precook and package meals and snacks is an example of

A) time management.
B) state of change.
C) environmental management.
D) alternative behaviors.

130. Free weight benches with barbells should accommodate

A) at least two spotters.
B) at least three spotters.
C) at least one spotter.
D) at least the person lifting the barbell.

131. What does the A stand for in the ABC model of behavior?

A) absolute
B) awards
C) antecedents
D) apathy

132. What do children tend to lack when starting a training program?

A) muscles
B) aerobic capacity
C) coordination
D) need of supervision

133. During clinical exercise testing protocols at a medical facility, it is the certified fitness professional's responsibility to

A) administer testing procedures under the guidance of a physician.
B) administer medical treatment and medical procedures to the client.
C) diagnose the client's symptoms based on the exercise test.
D) supervise the physician and staff during testing protocols.

134. If a relapse occurs, using positive self-talk to acknowledge successes is an example of which behavioral change tool?

A) cognitive coping
B) social support
C) relapse prevention
D) time management

135. The readiness-to-change theory differs from the other behavior change models, because it indicates _____ stages of change.

A) no
B) generalized
C) distinct
D) two

136. What should NOT be done during a hip sled?

A) bending the knees
B) raising the toes
C) locking the knees
D) pressing into the heels

137. A personal trainer's attire should be

    A) tasteful and modest fitness clothing.

    B) jeans and a t-shirt.

    C) tight and revealing.

    D) sweaty and worn.

138. Being able to _____ _____ is the best way to outline a plan of action to utilize session times effectively and efficiently.

    A) exercise first

    B) change behaviors

    C) set goals

    D) eat less

139. Which of the following techniques CANNOT be used to build persistence?

    A) create a network of excellence

    B) set goals using the SMART principle

    C) reward success

    D) create incentive programs

140. Proper maintenance and routine checking of fitness equipment can help prevent

    A) client dissatisfaction.

    B) environmental emergencies.

    C) negligence lawsuits.

    D) overtraining injuries.

141. Core exercises are classified into two sub categories: structural and _____.

    A) open

    B) assistance

    C) power

    D) static

142. Why is it important that fitness professionals obtain certification through a leading organization in the fitness industry?

    A) Trainers who are certified can make more money.

    B) Clients will often research the fitness professional's expertise and certifications.

    C) Trainers can guarantee client results with their certification.

    D) Certification is proof of the trainer's education.

143. Performing _____ stretching in a circuit can be a cardio warm-up.

    A) static

    B) passive

    C) dynamic

    D) active

144. How many spotters are needed for a dumbbell shoulder press?

    A) none

    B) 2

    C) 3

    D) 1

145. The body's response mechanism to absorbing too much physical stress in too short a time is called

    A) hypertension.

    B) hyperventilation.

    C) delayed onset muscle soreness.

    D) overtraining.

146. What method can assist the fitness professional in determining if a client is potentially overtraining?

   A) ask the client if he thinks he is overtraining

   B) ask one of the client's relatives for an opinion on whether the client is overtraining

   C) keep detailed records of the client's training outcomes and responses to training

   D) send the client to another fitness professional

147. What are the legal parameters in which all credentialed or licensed health professionals should work?

   A) scope of product

   B) legality of specialization

   C) scope of practice

   D) terms of work

148. What is an appropriate amount to increase cardiovascular training variables?

   A) 0.5 percent

   B) 10 percent

   C) 11 percent

   D) 15 percent

149. Which of the following is NOT a legal or ethical standard for personal trainers?

   A) denying culpability for personal actions

   B) maintaining accurate and honest notes for each client

   C) not discriminating based on race, gender, creed, age, ability, or sexual orientation

   D) complying with sexual harassment standards for both clients and peers

150. If a client has a muscle imbalance, what should she be directed to do in her warm-up?

   A) active stretching before static stretching

   B) SMR or foam roll before dynamic stretching

   C) static stretching before cardio warm-up

   D) SMR or foam roll before static stretching

1. **A) Correct.** The balance error scoring system requires the use of a spotter since the eyes are closed during portions of the test.

   B) Incorrect. The single-leg squat test does not require a spotter.

   C) Incorrect. The star excursion balance test does not require a spotter since the eyes remain open during the assessment.

   D) Incorrect. The overhead squat test does not require a spotter since both feet remain on the ground.

2. A) Incorrect. This is a function of the bones.

   B) Incorrect. This is a function of the bones.

   C) Incorrect. This is a function of the bones.

   D) Correct. Bones do NOT produce force for movement.

3. A) Incorrect. This refers to base of support.

   B) Incorrect. This does not accurately describe center of gravity.

   C) Correct. This is the definition of center of gravity.

   D) Incorrect. This is not an accurate representation of center of gravity.

4. A) Incorrect. This is when the palm is rotated toward the ground.

   B) Correct. This is the definition of supination.

   C) Incorrect. This occurs when a limb is pulled away from the midline of the body.

   D) Incorrect. This occurs as a joint angle is decreased through muscle contraction.

5. A) Incorrect. These do not assist the agonists.

   B) Incorrect. These prevent unwanted compensatory movement rather than assist in primary movement.

   C) Incorrect. These muscles help stabilize joints during exercises.

   D) Correct. This is the definition of synergists.

6. **A) Correct.** The waist-to-hip ratio measurement will identify individuals who are at a greater risk for disease.

   B) Incorrect. The Rockport walk test will not identify if individuals are at risk for disease.

   C) Incorrect. BMI measurements will not identify individuals who are at risk for disease since the BMI does not account for muscle mass.

   D) Incorrect. The balance error scoring system test assesses balance and will not identify individuals who are at a greater risk for disease.

7. **A) Correct.** The *t*-test is used to assess overall agility.

   B) Incorrect. The 1.5-mile run test is used to assess cardiorespiratory aerobic power.

   C) Incorrect. The three-minute step test is used to measure cardiorespiratory fitness and to determine how long it takes an individual to recover from short bouts of exercise.

   D) Incorrect. The Rockport walk test is used to measure aerobic capacity.

8. **A) Correct.** The higher the force applied, the more emphasis on muscular strength.

   B) Incorrect. Muscular endurance is not relevant to the force-velocity curve.

   C) Incorrect. Muscular power relies on a combination of force and velocity.

   D) Incorrect. Muscular speed relies heavily on velocity of movement.

9. A) Incorrect. The long jump test measures maximal horizontal jump distance.

   B) Correct. The reactive strength index test measures the body's reactive jump capacity and the stretch-shortening cycle effort.

C) Incorrect. The forty-yard dash is used to assess maximal speed.

D) Incorrect. The hexagon test is used to assess speed, agility, and quickness.

10. A) Incorrect. Kettlebells are considered free weights.

B) Incorrect. Dumbbells are considered free weights.

C) Incorrect. Sandbags are considered free weights.

D) Correct. A cardio machine is not portable; therefore, it is not considered a free weight.

11. A) Incorrect. Carbohydrates are consumed in relatively large quantities—hundreds of grams per day—to fuel metabolism and exercise, which makes them macronutrients.

B) Incorrect. Protein is a macronutrient and is required in the tens to over a hundred grams per day to maintain body structure and function.

C) Incorrect. Fat typically is consumed in tens of grams per day—about 30 percent of caloric intake—and is a major structural component of the body, comprising cell membranes and cushioning the organs. It is a macronutrient.

D) Correct. Vitamins are micronutrients; they are only required in small quantities, typically micrograms to milligrams per day.

12. A) Incorrect. Lactic acid does not cause DOMS.

B) Incorrect. Static stretching does not cause DOMS.

C) Correct. Micro-tears in the muscle fibers from resistance training cause DOMS.

D) Incorrect. Fit individuals can also experience DOMS.

13. A) Incorrect. Setting goals and planning will answer *how*.

B) Incorrect. This would be a negative response to a client.

C) Correct. This question will help a client uncover an intrinsic motivator.

D) Incorrect. This question will not help uncover intrinsic motivations.

14. **A) Correct.** Vitamin D regulates calcium and phosphate absorption in the intestine as well as their excretion by the kidneys; it also regulates mineral deposition and mobilization from bone.

B) Incorrect. Vitamin A deficiency does not manifest itself in bone effects.

C) Incorrect. Vitamin C deficiency can cause bone weakness due to decreased collagen in the bone, but it does not decrease bone mineralization.

D) Incorrect. Vitamin K is involved in bone formation, but problems in blood clotting show up well before bone problems caused by deficiency, which are rare.

15. A) Incorrect. Previous exercise experience is not found on the health history questionnaire.

B) Correct. General health information is found on the health history questionnaire.

C) Incorrect. The lifestyle questionnaire provides information about the client's lifestyle.

D) Incorrect. Information about the client's work history is not found on the health history questionnaire.

16. A) Incorrect. A machine leg extension is not a closed chain movement; a squat would be an example of a closed chain movement—with one or both legs on the floor.

B) Incorrect. A machine leg extension is not a core movement as it only focuses on one muscle group and a single joint motion, as opposed to several muscle groups and joints at a time.

C) Correct. In a machine leg extension, the machine allows both legs to lift at the same time, keeping the kinetic chain open.

D) Incorrect. A machine leg extension focuses on leg extension, which is a movement that falls in the sagittal plane of motion.

17. A) Incorrect. This will not likely elicit the neuroendocrine response to exercise.

B) Incorrect. This will not likely elicit the neuroendocrine response to exercise.

C) Incorrect. This is not an intense enough activity to elicit the neuroendocrine response to exercise.

D) Correct. Large muscle group, high-intensity exercise will elicit the neuroendocrine response to exercise.

18. A) Incorrect. 120/80 is an acceptable blood pressure reading.

B) Incorrect. 115/75 is a normal blood pressure reading.

C) Incorrect. 130/70 is a normal blood pressure reading.

D) Correct. 140/90 is a categorized as high blood pressure.

19. A) Incorrect. Knee flexion is incorrect.

B) Correct. These are the two actions of the quadriceps muscles.

C) Incorrect. Knee flexion and hip extension are both incorrect.

D) Incorrect. Hip extension is incorrect.

20. A) Incorrect. This is not true of many sports such as baseball, football, basketball, and hockey.

B) Incorrect. This is not true in many long-distance sports such as marathons, triathlons, long-distance swimming, and long-distance rowing.

C) Correct. The work-to-rest ratio should be designed and implemented based on the energy needs of the sport.

D) Incorrect. Cardiovascular exercise is equally as important in sports as resistance training.

21. A) Incorrect. This is an auto-immune inflammatory attack on the joints that causes joint degeneration.

B) Incorrect. This is inflammation of the joint.

C) Correct. This is the definition of osteoporosis.

D) Incorrect. This is an issue with posture due to muscular imbalance.

22. A) Incorrect. Marathoners benefit more from slow-twitch muscle fibers.

B) Incorrect. Such swimmers benefit more from slow-twitch muscle fibers.

C) Correct. Olympic sprinters require fast-twitch muscle fibers for improved performance.

D) Incorrect. Cross-country cyclists benefit more from slow-twitch muscle fibers.

23. A) Incorrect. A spotter cannot be used in a hip hinge motion.

B) Incorrect. Medicine ball slams are explosive exercises and therefore cannot use a spotter; the weight is not heavy enough.

C) Correct. Back-loaded squats, structural exercises, can use up to three spotters to ensure proper form.

D) Incorrect. Walking lunges are characterized by forward motion and cannot use a spotter.

24. A) Incorrect. The purpose of the medical clearance form is to determine if an individual should participate in an unsupervised, supervised, or medically supervised exercise program.

B) Correct. The lifestyle questionnaire will help identify a client's goals based on questions regarding the client's lifestyle and personal interests.

C) Incorrect. A body composition test will not accurately identify a client's goals.

D) Incorrect. A health history questionnaire will provide information on current and prior health.

25. A) Incorrect. The shoulders reveal upper crossed syndrome

B) Incorrect. The foot and ankle reveal pronation distortion syndrome.

C) Incorrect. The head and cervical spine reveal upper crossed syndrome.

D) Correct. The lumbo/pelvic/hip complex reveals lower crossed syndrome.

26. A) Incorrect. The lengthy aerobic demands as well as increased sweat losses associated with endurance exercise are more likely to cause an iron deficiency than strength training.

B) Incorrect. Male athletes are at lower risk than female athletes for iron deficiency since they tend to eat more meat and do not have menstrual iron losses.

C) Incorrect. As described in answer choice A, strength athletes are not at a high risk for iron-deficiency anemia.

D) Correct. Endurance athletes have higher iron requirements as well as higher iron losses. Female athletes have menstrual losses and also tend to consume less calories and meat than males; these can contribute to iron-deficiency anemia. Since iron from meat is the most bioavailable form, vegetarians are also at risk for iron-deficiency anemia, especially vegetarian endurance athletes.

27. A) Incorrect. Ladder drills are agility training.

B) Correct. Plyometrics uses short bursts of explosive motion to propel the body up or forward.

C) Incorrect. Running, swimming, or using a rowing machine for an extended period of time are all examples of cardio training.

D) Incorrect. Circuit training uses various exercises in a continuous sequence with minimal rest.

28. **A) Correct.** Typical mesocycles include multiple microcycles and last around six to twelve weeks.

B) Incorrect. This time period is too short.

C) Incorrect. This time period is too long and is more likely for a macrocycle.

D) Incorrect. This time period is far too long for a single mesocycle and the client will never reach peak performance.

29. A) Incorrect. Contractile proteins are major components of muscle fibers.

B) Incorrect. Enzymes are special types of proteins that catalyze reactions.

C) Incorrect. Many membrane receptors are proteins.

D) Correct. Cell membranes are composed primarily of phospholipids, not protein.

30. A) Incorrect. The compensation of the knees would be adducted or abducted.

B) Correct. The compensation of the feet from the anterior view is neither flattened nor externally rotated.

C) Incorrect. The compensation of the hips is anteriorly or posteriorly rotated.

D) Incorrect. The compensation of the head is tilted or rotated.

31. **A) Correct.** The 300-yard shuttle is used to measure anaerobic capacity.

B) Incorrect. The twelve-minute run assessment measures oxygen pathways for energy while running.

C) Incorrect. The three-minute step test measures submaximal aerobic fitness.

D) Incorrect. The 1.5-mile run test is used to measure an individual's aerobic power (cardiovascular endurance).

32. A) Incorrect. This is too soon.

B) Correct. After several weeks of resistance training, neuromuscular coordination is improved.

C) Incorrect. The benefits can be seen sooner than four weeks.

D) Incorrect. The benefits can be seen sooner than six weeks.

33. A) Incorrect. A mesocycle typically includes multiple microcycles.

B) Incorrect. A macrocycle includes the entire periodization.

C) **Correct.** A microcycle is the shortest cycle in a periodization.

D) Incorrect. The preparatory period typically involves mesocycles and microcycles.

34. A) **Correct.** Abnormal or disordered heart rhythms are known as arrhythmias.

B) Incorrect. This is part of the female athlete triad.

C) Incorrect. This is abnormally high blood pressure.

D) Incorrect. This is a hardening of the arteries.

35. A) Incorrect. How an individual moves is dynamic posture, not static posture.

B) Incorrect. Dynamic posture best represents alignment during movement.

C) **Correct.** Static posture is best represented when an individual is standing still.

D) Incorrect. Posture exhibited during exercise is dynamic posture.

36. A) Incorrect. This is the assessment that ensures that the content of the tests are relevant and appropriate.

B) Incorrect. This measures whether scores from similar assessments are related to the same outcome.

C) Incorrect. This is based on tests that measure what is intended.

D) **Correct.** This is the validity that is described in the question.

37. A) Incorrect. This statement is only partially true.

B) Incorrect. This describes a behavior modification technique.

C) Incorrect. Self-doubt is correct but it is only one aspect of this step in planning.

D) **Correct.** Managing fear and self-doubt is the goal of the belief step.

38. A) Incorrect. The Rockport walk test assesses cardiorespiratory endurance.

B) Incorrect. The push-up test is a muscular endurance test.

C) **Correct.** The hexagon test is used to assess speed, agility, and quickness.

D) Incorrect. The twelve-minute run test is used to assess cardiorespiratory endurance.

39. A) Incorrect. This is not the leading cause of preventable death according to the CDC.

B) Incorrect. This is not the leading cause of preventable death according to the CDC.

C) Incorrect. This is not the leading cause of preventable death according to the CDC.

D) **Correct.** This is the leading cause of preventable death according to the CDC.

40. A) **Correct.** The 300-yard shuttle test is used to measure anaerobic capacity.

B) Incorrect. The LEFT is used to measure agility in the sagittal and frontal plane.

C) Incorrect. The pro-agility test measures lateral speed and agility.

D) Incorrect. The *t*-test is used to assess overall agility while moving forward, laterally, and backward.

41. A) Incorrect. This assessment is used to check for optimal alignment.

B) Incorrect. This assessment is used to check for muscle symmetry.

C) **Correct.** This assessment is not used to check for overhead squat posturing.

D) Incorrect. This assessment is used to check for balanced muscle tone.

42. A) Incorrect. Stretch-release is the principle of static stretching.

B) **Correct.** In hold-relax, the stretching partner holds the stretch for 30 seconds and then allows the muscle to relax briefly before stretching again.

C) Incorrect. *Relax-breathe* is not a stretching sequence.

D) Incorrect. *Contract-contract* is not a stretching sequence.

43. A) Incorrect. The bench press test may not be appropriate for prenatal clients. In some situations, prenatal clients should avoid exercises in the supine position after they are twelve weeks into their pregnancy.

    B) Incorrect. The single squat may not be appropriate for prenatal clients as their center of gravity has changed due to pregnancy.

    C) **Correct.** The gait assessment would be the most appropriate assessment due to its low intensity.

    D) Incorrect. The forty-yard dash would not be appropriate as it measures maximal speed.

44. A) Incorrect. The radial pulse point is commonly used but not the brachial pulse point.

    B) Incorrect. The carotid pulse point is commonly used but not the brachial pulse point.

    C) Incorrect. The radial pulse point is commonly used but not the femoral pulse point.

    D) **Correct.** The carotid and radial pulse are the two most commonly used pulse points.

45. A) Incorrect. Muscle glycogen becomes important at middle distances.

    B) Incorrect. Intramuscular triglycerides become important at middle distances.

    C) **Correct.** These are the most readily available sources of energy and are first used in a sprint.

    D) Incorrect. Liver glycogen becomes important at long distances where muscle glycogen and blood glucose are depleted.

46. A) **Correct.** The pro-agility test measures lateral speed and agility.

    B) Incorrect. The barbell squat test measures lower body strength.

    C) Incorrect. The single-leg squat assessment tests dynamic flexibility.

    D) Incorrect. The push-up test is used to assess upper body muscular endurance.

47. A) **Correct.** This describes negative reinforcement.

    B) Incorrect. Finding a workout buddy is a demonstration of the social support technique.

    C) Incorrect. Creating a social media group would be considered a social support technique.

    D) Incorrect. Asking a friend or family member for support is one method in the social support technique.

48. A) **Correct.** The transversus abdominis is part of the stabilizer muscle system in the core.

    B) Incorrect. The hip flexors are part of the movement system of the core.

    C) Incorrect. The erector spinae is part of the movement system of the core.

    D) Incorrect. The abductor complex is part of the movement system of the core.

49. A) Incorrect. The DEXA scan is used to measure body fat percentage.

    B) **Correct.** Body mass index measurements do not measure body fat but determine if an individual's weight is appropriate for his or her height.

    C) Incorrect. Near-infrared interactance is used to measure body fat percentage.

    D) Incorrect. Air displacement plethysmography is used to measure body fat percentage.

50 A) Incorrect. Concurrent validity determines if scores are related to those of other acceptable tests of the same ability.

    B) Incorrect. Discriminant validity is the ability of a test to distinguish between two concepts and has shown low correlation between results.

    C) Incorrect. Content validity ensures that the testing being conducted covers all relevant component abilities of the test.

D) Correct. Face validity refers to a test that appears to measure what it is intended to measure.

51. A) Incorrect. The BMI formula takes height into account.

    B) Incorrect. The BMI formula takes height into account.

    C) Correct. Strength training builds lean muscle mass, which is a healthy kind of excess weight.

    D) Incorrect. For a sedentary individual, excess weight would likely be unhealthy fat, and BMI would be a measure of that.

52. A) Incorrect. This is not a method of checking the body's postural integrity.

    B) Incorrect. This is not a method of checking the body's postural integrity.

    C) Incorrect. This is not a method of checking the body's postural integrity.

    D) Correct. This is the system a personal trainer uses to check the posture of an individual.

53. **A) Correct.** This is the definition of scoliosis.

    B) Incorrect. This is excessive anterior curvature of the spine.

    C) Incorrect. This is decreased bone mineral density leading to bone brittleness.

    D) Incorrect. This is excessive posterior curvature of the spine.

54. A) Incorrect. Readiness for activity will be determined by answers given in the PAR-Q questionnaire.

    B) Incorrect. Medical problems will be discussed during the health history questionnaire.

    C) Incorrect. Medication taken by the client will be discussed during the health history or medical questionnaire.

    D) Correct. Stressors that may affect the client will be discussed during the lifestyle questionnaire.

55. A) Incorrect. With female clients, the thigh is measured, but the biceps and chest are not.

    B) Correct. The triceps, suprailium, and thigh are the three sites measured on female clients.

    C) Incorrect. The thigh and suprailium are measured, but the subscapular is not measured on female clients.

    D) Incorrect. The suprailium and thigh are measured on female clients; the biceps are not.

56. **A) Correct.** Time-bound goals keep a client motivated to meet a deadline.

    B) Incorrect. Challenging goals do not necessarily need a deadline.

    C) Incorrect. Proximal goals are small and progressive goals.

    D) Incorrect. Realistic goals are also progressive goals.

57. A) Incorrect. Fitness assessment is within a personal trainer's scope of practice.

    B) Incorrect. Program design is within a personal trainer's scope of practice.

    C) Correct. Massage therapy is not within a personal trainer's scope of practice.

    D) Incorrect. Goal-setting is within a personal trainer's scope of practice.

58. **A) Correct.** The dynamic warm-up should be specific to the exercise performed in the workout.

    B) Incorrect. Flexibility is improved by static stretching, which should be performed after the workout.

    C) Incorrect. Specific movement preparation will better prepare the body for specific movements. A basic general warm-up may not adequately prepare the body for the excess stress of the workout and may lead to injury or poor performance.

    D) Incorrect. Exercises for muscular power should be performed during the workout, not the warm-up.

59.

A) Incorrect. The bench press test would not be appropriate for this goal.

B) Incorrect. The hexagon test would not be appropriate for this goal.

C) Correct. The Rockport walk test would be the most appropriate test for the goal of lowering a client's blood pressure.

D) Incorrect. The three-hundred-yard shuttle test would not be appropriate for this goal.

60.

A) Correct. This test measures one's ability to change directions and stabilize the body at high speeds.

B) Incorrect. This test measures an individual's agility while moving laterally, forward, and backward.

C) Incorrect. This test measures lateral speed and agility.

D) Incorrect. This test is used to measure total body bilateral power.

61.

A) Incorrect. Body control is synonymous with form.

B) Correct. Breath is a key component of exercise technique and lifting heavy loads.

C) Incorrect. Flexibility is important but not necessary when adding heavy weight loads.

D) Incorrect. While a positive outlook is important, it is not an athlete's primary focus when he or she is lifting heavy loads.

62.

A) Incorrect. A supine position requires the body to be totally flat.

B) Incorrect. A sitting position is not the correct starting position.

C) Correct. In a semi-supine position, the body is face up on the floor with the knees bent and feet planted on the floor.

D) Incorrect. In a prone position, the body is lying face down.

63.

A) Correct. This compensation can be viewed anteriorly.

B) Incorrect. This compensation can be viewed posteriorly.

C) Incorrect. This compensation can be viewed posteriorly.

D) Incorrect. This compensation can be viewed posteriorly.

64.

A) Incorrect. Love is not being described in this statement.

B) Incorrect. This is not the correct description of fear.

C) Incorrect. This is not the correct description of locus of control.

D) Correct. This statement accurately describes persistence.

65.

A) Incorrect. The terms *power*, *muscle*, and *matter* do not represent progressive fitness levels.

B) Incorrect. *Hard* is not a fitness level.

C) Correct. The terms *stabilization*, *strength*, and *power* represent three fitness levels.

D) Incorrect. *Body* is not correct.

66.

A) Correct. Structural exercises load the spine, the main postural component of the body to increase strength.

B) Incorrect. Power exercises are core exercises, but they are not load bearing and typically utilize reactive motions to increase force production.

C) Incorrect. Agility exercises typically do not use any weight and focus on agility through footwork and deceleration.

D) Incorrect. Assistance exercises are not core exercises and recruit single joint action and small muscle groups.

67.

A) Incorrect. The drawing-in maneuver does activate the core.

B) Incorrect. The drawing-in maneuver maintains neutral posturing.

C) Incorrect. The drawing-in maneuver is used for all core exercises.

D) Correct. The drawing-in maneuver does not stretch the hips.

68.

A) Incorrect. Agility is the body's ability to accelerate, decelerate, and change directions quickly while maintaining stability.

B) Incorrect. Force is the body's ability to use power to do any muscle contraction.

C) **Correct.** Speed is the body's ability to use force and move in one direction as quickly as possible.

D) Incorrect. Power is synonymous with force production.

69. A) Incorrect. The overhead squat test is used to assess neuromuscular efficiency.

B) Incorrect. The overhead squat test is used to assess functional strength.

C) **Correct.** The single-leg squat test is used to assess unilateral balance.

D) Incorrect. The overhead squat is used to test dynamic flexibility.

70. A) Incorrect. Core exercises typically recruit large muscle groups and have multiple joint motions.

B) Incorrect. Open kinetic chain exercises do activate smaller muscle groups, but they are not used for just rehabilitative purposes.

C) Incorrect. PNF stretching is stretching used for rehabilitative purposes and typically requires assistance from another person.

D) **Correct.** Assistance exercises are used for rehabilitative purposes; they isolate a specific, smaller muscle group.

71. A) Incorrect. There are ways to progress a single-leg squat.

B) Incorrect. This would be a regression of the same exercise.

C) **Correct.** Adding weight to the exercise will increase the intensity and be a progression.

D) Incorrect. A new exercise would not be a progression of the same exercise.

72. A) Incorrect. Neuromuscular efficiency only addresses the relationship between the nervous system and the muscular system.

B) Incorrect. The term *progressive system* refers to the exercise training continuum, not the body systems.

C) **Correct.** The term *kinetic chain* refers to the connection among all three movement systems.

D) Incorrect. *Postural balance* is not a specific term.

73. A) Incorrect. Uncontrollable metabolic disease is a relative contraindication.

B) **Correct.** Symptomatic heart failure is an absolute contraindication.

C) Incorrect. A musculoskeletal disorder is a relative contraindication.

D) Incorrect. A history of heart illness is a relative contraindication.

74. A) Incorrect. Lower back pain does not require a client to see a medical professional.

B) Incorrect. Anterior knee pain does not require immediate medical attention.

C) **Correct.** A client who has had a recent complication due to cardiac disease must be referred to a medical professional before the assessment may begin.

D) Incorrect. A client who does not feel well generally does not need an immediate medical referral.

75. A) Incorrect. Dynamic stretching helps to improve muscle elasticity and blood flow prior to exercise.

B) **Correct.** Static stretching elicits an elongation of the muscle through a static holding of a stretch.

C) Incorrect. Self-myofascial release involves using tools to compress adhesions in the fascia that surrounds muscle bodies.

D) Incorrect. The dynamic warm-up does not involve static stretching to elongate muscle.

76. A) Incorrect. The excessive fatigue associated with this volume and load range can negate performance during the season.

B) **Correct.** The off-season should include a period of muscular endurance development because athletic performance will not be hindered during competition.

C) Incorrect. Excessive fatigue from muscular endurance training should be avoided during the competitive period because it can cause deleterious effects on performance.

D) Incorrect. The second transition period should involve recreational activities and a break from resistance training protocols.

77. A) Incorrect. Static stretching can limit strength and power output, causing poor performance and potential injury.

B) Incorrect. Static stretching can harm power exercise performance such as plyometrics.

C) Incorrect. Cardiovascular exercise should follow the same warm-up protocol as resistance training.

D) **Correct.** Static stretching should be implemented in a flexibility program after the muscles have been warmed up and exercised to elongate the muscles.

78. A) Incorrect. This is a set.

B) Incorrect. This is not the definition of a repetition.

C) Incorrect. This is not the definition of a repetition.

D) **Correct.** The performance of an exercise one time through its full range of motion is a repetition.

79. A) Incorrect. Static stretching should not be part of the warm-up.

B) Incorrect. Single-muscle group exercises and plyometrics should not be performed until after the warm-up is complete.

C) **Correct.** These three items should always be included in the warm-up process for ideal preparation.

D) Incorrect. Although dynamic stretching and foam rolling may be beneficial to the field hockey player, PNF stretching may inhibit the player's performance during the workout.

80. A) Incorrect. Horizontal loading refers to performing multiple sets of a single exercise with intermittent rest periods.

B) Incorrect. Single set refers to performing one set of each exercise during a workout.

C) Incorrect. Interval training refers to using a timer to determine the work-to-rest ratio rather than repetitions.

D) **Correct.** Vertical loading is a form of circuit training that loads different muscles per exercise to minimize rest.

81. A) Incorrect. Maintaining training loads will not elicit the overload effect.

B) **Correct.** A gradual progression of training loads will elicit the overload effect.

C) Incorrect. Decreasing training loads does not follow the principle of overload.

D) Incorrect. Rapidly increasing training loads can cause overuse injuries and prevent improvements.

82. A) Incorrect. Flexibility is not greatly improved by either of these training techniques.

B) Incorrect. Power exercises are high intensity.

C) Incorrect. Muscular endurance exercises are lower intensity.

D) **Correct.** Since technique is important with power exercises, they should be performed before the muscles suffer from fatigue and performance suffers.

83. A) Incorrect. This refers to the training frequency.

B) Incorrect. This is the type of exercise the client is performing.

C) **Correct.** RPE stands for Rating of Perceived Exertion, or how difficult the client feels the activity is on a scale of one through ten.

D) Incorrect. This is not what the RPE scale represents.

84.

A) Incorrect. Seven points of contact is appropriate for a supine position and would include the right calf and left calf.

B) Incorrect. Three points of contact refers to a neutral standing position—the head, mid-back, and glutes would touch the wall.

C) Incorrect. There are no body positions that require four points of contact.

D) Correct. The five points of contact in a semi-supine position are at the head, shoulders, glutes, right foot, and left foot.

85.

A) Correct. The ABC model of behavior helps a person identify triggers for unwanted and desirable behaviors.

B) Incorrect. Obsessions are not a focus of this model.

C) Incorrect. Irritants can be considered a negative trigger, but not a positive one.

D) Incorrect. Successes can be considered a product of using this model.

86.

A) Correct. Increases in training load are associated with an obligatory decrease in volume to avoid overuse or overtraining.

B) Incorrect. Decreasing loads are associated with increasing volumes.

C) Incorrect. Maintaining load with a decrease in volume will reduce the chances of the program causing a progressive overload on the muscles. The client won't get the desired results.

D) Incorrect. Both training variables should change when either of them changes.

87.

A) Incorrect. Testosterone is a type of anabolic hormone.

B) Incorrect. IGF is a type of anabolic hormone.

C) Incorrect. Epinephrine is a type of hormone associated with environmental stressors.

D) Correct. The two hormone types associated with exercise are anabolic and catabolic.

88.

A) Incorrect. This is the definition of exercise regression.

B) Incorrect. This is called peaking.

C) Incorrect. This is the principle of progression.

D) Correct. A training plateau is when the client is not seeing any benefit from the exercise program.

89.

A) Incorrect. While quickness and agility are connected, agility is the body's ability to accelerate and decelerate more so than reacting to a direction change.

B) Correct. Quickness is the body's ability to react to changing direction.

C) Incorrect. *Readiness* is not a term that describes an exercise function.

D) Incorrect. Stabilization is the body's ability to utilize the core efficiently.

90.

A) Correct. This network is called the allied healthcare continuum.

B) Incorrect. The term *training continuum* describes a progressive system in exercise technique.

C) Incorrect. While those in the network are considered health professionals, this is not the proper name of the network.

D) Incorrect. The term *health maintenance professionals* is not correct.

91.

A) Incorrect. Strength training is also known as resistance training.

B) Incorrect. Force training is not a type of training.

C) Incorrect. Quickness training is also known as reactive training.

D) Correct. Plyometrics is sometimes referred to as *power training* because it uses explosive movements.

92.

A) Incorrect. The transversus abdominis are stabilizing muscles.

B) Correct. The latissimus dorsi is the prime mover for the lateral pulldown.

C) Incorrect. The anterior deltoids are synergistic muscles for the lateral pulldown.

D) Incorrect. The legs are not a focus in a lateral pulldown.

93. A) Incorrect. Using the ABC model of behavior to identify triggers is an example of relapse prevention and recovery plans.

   B) **Correct.** Planning a weekly menu and a shopping list is an example of time management, not relapse prevention and recovery plans.

   C) Incorrect. Not focusing on fault is an example of relapse prevention and recovery plans.

   D) Incorrect. Relapse prevention and recovery plans can include creating contingency plans.

94. A) Incorrect. The program is incomplete and missing warm-up, cooldown, and cardiovascular training.

   B) Incorrect. The program is incomplete and missing warm-up, cooldown, and resistance training.

   C) Incorrect. The program is incomplete and missing warm-up, cooldown, resistance training, and cardiovascular training.

   D) **Correct.** This program includes all of the major components of a workout.

95. A) Incorrect. A macrocycle includes off-season training as well.

   B) **Correct.** The macrocycle encompasses the entire training periodization.

   C) Incorrect. A macrocycle includes in-season training as well.

   D) Incorrect. A macrocycle includes all preparatory, transition, competition, and second transition periods.

96. A) Incorrect. Diet journaling is a self-monitoring tool to modify behavior.

   B) Incorrect. Activity tracking is another example of a self-monitoring tool.

   C) **Correct.** This is an example of the rewarding technique for behavior modification.

D) Incorrect. Incorporating weekly weigh-ins would be considered a self-monitoring tool.

97. A) **Correct.** Only 7 percent of communication is through verbal communication.

   B) Incorrect. The figure of 10 percent is not accurate.

   C) Incorrect. Fifty-five percent of our communication is commonly attributed to our body language.

   D) Incorrect. Vocal quality makes up 38 percent of our communication.

98. A) Incorrect. It is impossible to peak throughout the entirety of a program.

   B) Incorrect. If the client peaks at the start, then there is no goal to reach with the program.

   C) **Correct.** The trainer should develop the periodization to have the client peak just prior to competitions or major events during the season.

   D) Incorrect. Peak performance is safe as long as the program does not intend to maintain this high intensity for too long. After peak performance is reached, maintenance training can begin, or an active rest can be taken following the completion of competition.

99. A) Incorrect. The maintenance phase is only half of the correct answer.

   B) Incorrect. The action phase is only half of the correct answer.

   C) **Correct.** Action and maintenance are the phases that will require behavior modification tools.

   D) Incorrect. Neither of these phases requires behavior modification tools.

100. A) Incorrect. Outdoor temperatures may be extreme and cause issues with overheating.

   B) Incorrect. Exercising in cold temperatures can cause issues with thermoregulation as well.

   C) **Correct.** Proper hydration is important because it helps children and adolescents to thermoregulate their body temperatures.

D) Incorrect. Exercise indoors can involve extreme temperatures as well.

101. **A)** **Correct.** Muscular power exercises that involve jumping increase the stress placed on the joints from impact and should be avoided.

B) Incorrect. Muscular endurance exercises will benefit obese individuals and cause little joint stress.

C) Incorrect. Muscular strength training benefits obese clients and does not necessarily cause excessive joint stress.

D) Incorrect. Muscular hypertrophy exercises will help to reduce body fat and increase lean mass, overall decreasing body weight and reducing stress.

102. A) Incorrect. This is too many repetitions and may cause fatigue before beginning.

B) Incorrect. This is not enough repetitions to adequately warm up the client.

C) Incorrect. This is a broad range and still too many repetitions, potentially fatiguing the client.

D) **Correct.** About five repetitions per warm-up exercise is adequate.

103. A) Incorrect. The client can benefit from other modes of aerobic exercise including running.

B) Incorrect. The client can benefit from other modes of aerobic exercise including these two.

C) **Correct.** For general health benefits, the mode of aerobic exercise does not matter and whatever modes the client prefers should be implemented.

D) Incorrect. For improvements to cardiovascular and respiratory fitness, which are important general health benefits, aerobic exercise is required.

104. A) Incorrect. This would be a progression of the exercise.

B) Incorrect. This would be a progression of the exercise.

C) Incorrect. This is a different exercise at a similar intensity.

D) **Correct.** A wall sit or wall slide exercise removes the stability required from the core and makes the exercise easier. It is a regression.

105. A) Incorrect. It is more appropriate to work opposing muscles on a superset. These exercises use the same primary muscles.

B) Incorrect. It is more appropriate to work opposing muscles on a superset.

C) **Correct.** A push-and-pull or pull-and-push superset is most appropriate.

D) Incorrect. Both of these exercises are push exercises working the same primary muscles.

106. A) Incorrect. Linear periodization does not implement three different muscular training phases in a microcycle.

B) **Correct.** This is an example of an undulating microcycle.

C) Incorrect. Regression refers to a decrease in exercise difficulty due to physical limitations.

D) Incorrect. The program is not necessarily dangerous if the client has been properly progressed.

107. A) Incorrect. The term *transitional* does not describe any type of fitness equipment.

B) Incorrect. Cardio equipment is non-portable and focuses on aerobic training only.

C) **Correct.** Functional equipment is portable and can be used for various types of training.

D) Incorrect. While the stability ball and resistance tubes are used for advanced controlled instability and strength training, a sandbag is used in explosive movements.

108. A) Incorrect. A program that focuses mainly on the upper body will not help to reduce chronic back pain.

B) **Correct.** Core strengthening and improving flexibility (especially in the hamstrings) can help to limit chronic back pain and should be the focus of the training program.

C) Incorrect. Lower body resistance training will not reduce lower back pain.

D) Incorrect. Avoiding the problem all together will only weaken the client and could potentially make things worse.

109. A) Incorrect. The assessment would take place after the initial connections.

B) Correct. Building a connection through agreement and similarity will initiate trust.

C) Incorrect. Using positive body language is an important aspect of communication, but it is not the first step in building client relationships

D) Incorrect. A high five and a smile are both non-verbal communication.

110. A) Incorrect. The first transition period is between the preparatory period and competitive period.

B) Incorrect. These are not the periods; they are the cycles.

C) Incorrect. The order is incorrect.

D) Correct. The preparatory period is first, followed by the first transition period, then the competitive period, and finally the second transition period.

111. **A) Correct.** These forms are used by fitness professionals to ensure they have taken all measures to improve client safety prior to exercise, to inform the client, and to ensure the trainer has the client's consent to begin training.

B) Incorrect. A client's hobbies may help in designing an exercise plan, but they will not minimize risk, and a bloodwork form is beyond the fitness professional's scope of practice.

C) Incorrect. The bloodwork form is beyond the fitness professional's scope of practice.

D) Incorrect. The fitness assessment should not be performed until all forms are completed and signed.

112. A) Incorrect. Nodding indicates positive body language.

B) Incorrect. Leaning forward is another way to indicate a positive body language.

C) Correct. Wringing hands is a negative body language indicator.

D) Incorrect. A firm handshake also indicates positive body language.

113. A) Incorrect. Though plyometrics do increase muscular power, they may place dangerous forces on the already overstressed joints of overweight individuals.

B) Incorrect. This is an opinion of the client and not relevant to the question.

C) Incorrect. They are in the category of higher intensity exercises and can be difficult for many people.

D) Correct. The force from landing after a plyometric jump exercise places excessive stress on the joints of the ankles, knees, and hips, and may be dangerous for individuals who are overweight or obese.

114. A) Incorrect. Vocal tone is non-verbal and words are verbal.

B) Incorrect. Body language is non-verbal and singing skills are neither verbal nor non-verbal.

C) Correct. Vocal tone and body language are both types of non-verbal communication.

D) Incorrect. Words are verbal communication and body language is non-verbal.

115. A) Incorrect. People in the preparation phase have a moderate self-efficacy but may still feel their locus of control is external.

B) Correct. People in the precontemplation phase have both a low self-efficacy and an external locus of control.

C) Incorrect. People in the action phase have grown their self-efficacy to a moderate level and are shifting from an external locus of control to an internal locus of control.

D) Incorrect. People in the termination phase have grown their self-efficacy maximally and have shifted into an internal locus of control.

116. A) Incorrect. Finger tapping is an indicator of negative body language.

B) **Correct.** Tall posture is a positive body language indicator.

C) Incorrect. Shifting eyes is also a negative body language indicator.

D) Incorrect. Arms crossed is another negative body language indicator.

117. A) Incorrect. Static stretching should happen in the middle of the warm-up.

B) Incorrect. PNF stretching should come in the middle of the warm-up, in lieu of static stretching if rehab is needed.

C) **Correct.** Dynamic stretching should be done at the end of the warm-up to target the muscle groups that will be worked during a workout.

D) Incorrect. SMR stretching is done after the general cardio warm-up if needed.

118. A) Incorrect. Standards of professionalism are included in the code of ethics for personal trainers.

B) Incorrect. The code of ethics for personal trainers includes standards for confidentiality.

C) **Correct.** Standards for friendship are not included in the code of ethics for personal trainers.

D) Incorrect. The code of ethics for personal trainers includes standards for business practices.

119. A) Incorrect. Facial expressions are body language.

B) Incorrect. Vocal quality is body language.

C) **Correct.** Spoken words are verbal communication.

D) Incorrect. Posture is body language.

120. A) Incorrect. Enthusiasm is the only one of the three attributes described correctly.

B) **Correct.** Confidence, enthusiasm, and professionalism are the three attributes a trainer should personify when meeting with a client.

C) Incorrect. Confidence is the only one of the three attributes described correctly.

D) Incorrect. None of these are among the three attributes described in the text.

121. A) Incorrect. Decrease in weight causes decrease in intensity.

B) Incorrect. Increase in volume causes decrease in weight and therefore decrease in intensity.

C) **Correct.** Increase in weight causes an increase in intensity.

D) Incorrect. Increase in repetitions is similar to increase in volume, causing a decrease in intensity.

122. A) Incorrect. A professional trainer would NOT wear khaki pants or jeans.

B) **Correct.** Tasteful athletic attire is appropriate for a professional trainer.

C) Incorrect. Revealing athletic attire is NOT appropriate for a professional trainer to wear.

D) Incorrect. Strong cologne or perfume is NOT appropriate for a professional trainer.

123. A) **Correct.** Active listening uses both verbal and non-verbal communication.

B) Incorrect. Body language is non-verbal communication.

C) Incorrect. Hopefully the trainer is empathetic and building a rapport with the client, but neither of these would be possible without verbal and non-verbal communication, so this is not the best answer. It is certain that verbal and non-verbal communication are occurring during active listening.

D) Incorrect. These are categories of exercises, not communication.

124. A) Incorrect. Although this is positive body language, it might not be an appropriate response.

B) Incorrect. Hugging is one type of empathetic body language, but it might not be an appropriate response to the client's statement.

C) Incorrect. This would be a negative response to a client.

D) Correct. Repeating key elements of a client's statement indicates active listening.

125. A) Incorrect. One year is not the correct renewal requirement.

B) Incorrect. Four years is not the correct renewal requirement for a personal training certification.

C) Incorrect. Six years is not correct.

D) Correct. A personal training certification needs to be renewed every two years.

126. A) Correct. Stimulus control is a behavior modification tool to facilitate a change of habits.

B) Incorrect. Socio-ecological theory is considered a behavioral change model.

C) Incorrect. Self-monitoring does not fit the description provided.

D) Incorrect. Locus of control is not a tool to bring about behavior change.

127. A) Incorrect. Setting reasonable goals to inhibit the possibility of unreasonable results cannot be considered self-monitoring.

B) Correct. Setting reasonable and attainable goals is an example of cognitive coping.

C) Incorrect. The description provided is not an example of rewarding.

D) Incorrect. Setting reasonable and attainable goals is positive, and is not an example of negative reinforcement.

128. A) Correct. A trainer must be realistic to help manage a client's expectations.

B) Incorrect. A trainer is not perfect and doesn't always have to be right,

although all trainers should strive to provide their clients with correct information.

C) Incorrect. A trainer should try not to make negative statements to their clients.

D) Incorrect. A trainer should not make a habit of spending time with clients outside of the sessions.

129. A) Correct. Preparing meals and snacks ahead of time is an example of the time-management technique.

B) Incorrect. The state-of-change theory does not include activities such as setting aside time for preparing meals in advance.

C) Incorrect. The task as described is not an example of environmental management.

D) Incorrect. Setting aside time for a task such as meal preparation is not an example of alternative behaviors.

130. A) Incorrect. Two spotters is too few.

B) Correct. There should be room for at least three spotters at a free weight barbell bench.

C) Incorrect. One spotter is not enough for a free weight bench.

D) Incorrect. There must be room for the lifter and at least three spotters.

131. A) Incorrect. The A in the ABC acronym does not stand for *absolute*.

B) Incorrect. The A in the acronym does not stand for *awards*.

C) Correct. The A in the ABC acronym stands for *antecedents*.

D) Incorrect. *Apathy* is not the correct answer.

132. A) Incorrect. All human beings have muscles.

B) Incorrect. Aerobic capacity is not typically an issue in children.

C) Correct. Children tend to lack the same coordination as adults.

D) Incorrect. Children should always be supervised during training sessions.

133. A) **Correct.** The certified fitness professional may administer the test under the guidance of the physician supervising the clinical team.

B) Incorrect. Medical treatment and procedures are the responsibility of the supervising physician.

C) Incorrect. Diagnosing symptoms is the responsibility of the supervising physician.

D) Incorrect. The certified fitness professional does not supervise the physician during testing procedures.

134. A) Incorrect. The activity as described is not an example of cognitive coping.

B) Incorrect. Self-talk is not part of social support.

C) **Correct.** Using positive self-talk to acknowledge successes is an example of the relapse prevention tool.

D) Incorrect. Time management does not include positive self-talk to acknowledge success.

135. A) Incorrect. The theory indicates six distinct stages of change.

B) Incorrect. The stages are specific, not generalized.

C) **Correct.** There are six distinct stages of change to indicate progressions.

D) Incorrect. There are six stages, not two.

136. A) Incorrect. It is necessary to bend the knees to complete a rep.

B) Incorrect. While this is not a part of a rep, raising the toes can be added to a repetition to incorporate the calves.

C) **Correct.** Locking the knees could cause a serious injury.

D) Incorrect. It is necessary to press into the heels to complete the repetitions properly.

137. A) **Correct.** A professional trainer should wear tasteful and modest attire that is representative of the fitness industry.

B) Incorrect. A professional trainer should wear attire appropriate for the fitness industry.

C) Incorrect. The attire of a professional trainer should be tasteful and modest.

D) Incorrect. A personal trainer's attire should be clean and appear professional to clients.

138. A) Incorrect. A person should not start an exercise plan until he or she has set goals.

B) Incorrect. While changing behavior is a goal of an exercise regimen, it is not how one begins a regimen.

C) **Correct.** Setting goals is an ideal way to start an effective exercise program so that sessions are used most efficiently.

D) Incorrect. Eating less is a product of setting goals.

139. A) Incorrect. Creating a network of excellence is one technique that can be used to build persistence.

B) **Correct.** This is not a technique for building persistence.

C) Incorrect. Rewarding success is among the techniques that can be used to build persistence.

D) Incorrect. Incentive programs can be used to build persistence.

140. A) Incorrect. Client dissatisfaction could be related to a number of issues.

B) Incorrect. Environmental emergencies typically are unavoidable, but emergency action plans can limit liability.

C) **Correct.** One potential source of negligence lawsuits is equipment breakdown and the resultant injuries. This risk can be reduced with routine equipment maintenance.

D) Incorrect. Overtraining injuries are not typically due to faulty equipment.

141. A) Incorrect. This is not a subcategory of core exercises.

B) Incorrect. This is the main classification of core exercises, not a subcategory.

C) **Correct.** Power exercises use multiple muscle groups and joint motions, but are not load-bearing, like structural.

D) Incorrect. This is a form of stretching.

142. A) Incorrect. Certification through leading organizations does not guarantee more money.

B) **Correct.** Clients who are thorough will research a fitness professional to make sure he or she has expertise in the field.

C) Incorrect. Certifications cannot guarantee client results.

D) Incorrect. Fitness certifications are not necessarily proof of higher education or training, although certified professionals have often obtained both.

143. A) Incorrect. Static stretching is a technique that uses an implement to hold the leg in place.

B) Incorrect. Passive stretching is not a cardio warm-up.

C) **Correct.** Dynamic stretching includes stretches that are more intense and utilize full range of motion, so when they are performed in a circuit, they could be a challenging cardio warm-up.

D) Incorrect. Active stretching is indeed a type of stretching that uses slow and controlled movements to increase range of motion, but it would not be challenging for a cardio warm-up.

144. A) Incorrect. Spotting requires at least one person.

B) Incorrect. A dumbbell shoulder press requires one spotter.

C) Incorrect. A dumbbell shoulder press requires one spotter.

D) **Correct.** One spotter is required behind the lifter, supporting the wrists.

145. A) Incorrect. Hypertension refers to high blood pressure.

B) Incorrect. Hyperventilation is an increased respiration rate.

C) Incorrect. Delayed onset muscle soreness is the normal physiological response related to micro-tears in the muscle fibers, causing acute muscular soreness.

D) **Correct.** The definition provided describes overtraining.

146. A) Incorrect. The client may not know the signs and symptoms of overtraining, or may give an inaccurate response.

B) Incorrect. The client's relatives may not know the signs and symptoms of overtraining.

C) **Correct.** Keeping accurate records of the client's progress means the trainer can consult data to determine whether the client is overtraining. There are often physiological and psychological symptoms associated with overtraining.

D) Incorrect. Another fitness professional meeting the client for the first time might consider the client's abilities normal.

147. A) Incorrect. The legal parameters are not called scope of product.

B) Incorrect. Legality of specialization is not the proper name for the legal parameters.

C) **Correct.** Scope of practice is the term that describes the legal parameters within which credentialed or licensed health professionals must work.

D) Incorrect. Terms of work is not the proper name.

148. A) Incorrect. This amount of training increase is too little to elicit an overload effect and training progression.

B) **Correct.** The cardiovascular training variables should not be increased by more than 10% from workout to workout.

C) Incorrect. This increase is too much and may cause overtraining.

D) Incorrect. This increase is too much and may cause overtraining.

149. A) **Correct.** Accepting responsibility for one's actions is not necessarily considered a legal or ethical issue, but it is a standard that a professional trainer should maintain.

B)   Incorrect. Maintaining accurate notes on each client is an ethical standard for personal trainers.

C)   Incorrect. This is a legal or ethical standard. Personal trainers must not discriminate based on race, gender, creed, age, ability, or sexual orientation.

D)   Incorrect. Complying with sexual harassment standards is a legal or ethical standard for personal trainers.

150. A)   Incorrect. General warm-up and SMR should come before static stretching.

B)   Incorrect. Dynamic stretching should be after static stretching.

C)   Incorrect. Cardio warm-up should come before static stretching.

D)   **Correct.** SMR is ideal to do before static stretching to ensure the loosening of muscle knots.

THREE: Practice Test Three

READ THE QUESTION, AND THEN CHOOSE THE MOST CORRECT ANSWER.

1. The biological hierarchy from the largest structure to the smallest structure is:

   A) organism, organ, organ system, tissue, cell.

   B) organism, organ system, organ, tissue, cell.

   C) organ system, organism, tissue, organ, cell.

   D) cell, tissue, organ, organ system, organism.

2. The heart is

   A) a cell.

   B) a tissue.

   C) an organ system.

   D) an organ.

3. Exhale on the _____ of the exercise.

   A) hold point or isometric movement

   B) exertion point or concentric movement

   C) extension point or eccentric movement

   D) sticking point or failure

4. What is criterion-referenced validity?

   A) the extent to which the test score corresponds with future performance

   B) the measure of the degree of consistency or repeatability of a test

   C) the extent to which test scores are related to an outcome with some other test of the same ability

   D) the degree to which a test measures what it is supposed to measure

5. What are the six phases in the readiness-to-change model?

   A) specific, challenging, attainable, measurable, proximal, inspirational

   B) environmental management, alternative behaviors, reward, social support, cognitive coping, relapse prevention

   C) precontemplation, contemplation, preparation, action, maintenance, termination

   D) individual, introvert, interpersonal, organizational, community, public policy

6. In order for a test to be reliable, which characteristics must the test display?

A) The test must be able to distinguish between two different concepts.

B) The test score must correspond with future performance.

C) The test must measure what it is designed to measure.

D) The test must deliver the same score or result.

7. When observing an individual during the static postural assessment, which position should be observed at the shoulder joint from the lateral view?

A) level, not elevated or rounded

B) neutral position, not flexed or extended

C) normal kyphotic curve

D) neutral position, not tilted or rotated

8. What is the difference between kyphosis and lordosis of the spine?

A) Kyphosis refers to excessive posterior curvature of the spine; lordosis is anterior.

B) Kyphosis refers to excessive anterior curvature of the spine; lordosis is posterior.

C) Kyphosis refers to excessive lateral curvature of the spine; lordosis is anterior.

D) The two terms are interchangeable.

9. Which joint allows for the most freedom of movement?

A) biaxial joints

B) hinge joints

C) saddle joints

D) ball-and-socket joints

10. Which of the following is the most energy-dense macronutrient?

A) carbohydrates

B) sugars

C) fats

D) protein

11. Regression refers to

A) the gradual increase in exercise intensity over the course of a periodized training program.

B) reducing the intensity of an exercise due to physical limitation or poor technique.

C) performing an exercise for one full range of motion.

D) the downward movement phase during the repetition of an exercise.

12. Through what organizations can a fitness specialist obtain CPR, AED, and first-aid training?

A) the American College of Sports Medicine (ACSM)

B) a local hospital

C) the same organization that provides personal trainers' insurance

D) the American Heart Association (AHA), OSHA, or the Red Cross

13. If asked about a specific dietary supplement recommendation, a fitness professional can respond if

A) he feels like it.

B) the personal trainer has personally taken the supplement and had positive results.

C) the fitness professional has personally taken it and had negative results.

D) the fitness professional has an additional nutrition certification.

14. Bone mineral density is developed more easily at what point in life?

A) adulthood

B) childhood

C) any age

D) advanced age

15. Which muscles are considered Type I muscles?

A) power muscles

B) weak muscles

C) postural muscles

D) leg muscles

16. Which of the following is the definition of *volume* as it refers to a training program?

A) the amount of weight lifted for a single repetition

B) the act of performing a specific number of repetitions through their full range of motion

C) the principle that involves gradually increasing the difficulty to elicit muscular adaptation over the course of the periodization

D) the total number of sets multiplied by the number of repetitions of a particular exercise

17. What should the fitness professional do with malfunctioning equipment?

A) place signage indicating the equipment is *Out of Order*, or remove the equipment from the fitness center floor

B) inform clientele upon their arrival to the facility that the equipment is not working properly

C) inform clientele about the equipment if the trainer sees a client using the equipment

D) disassemble the piece of equipment

18. Which group of vitamins participates in energy metabolism?

A) fat-soluble vitamins

B) antioxidant vitamins

C) most of the B vitamins

D) folate and B-12

19. During the static postural assessment, which kinetic chain checkpoints are analyzed?

A) the knees, shoulder, and head

B) the feet and knees

C) the foot/ankle, knees, lumbo/pelvic/hip complex, shoulders, and head

D) the shoulder and head

20. The precursor to osteoporosis is called

A) bone mineral density.

B) lordosis.

C) scoliosis.

D) osteopenia.

21. Body language encompasses all the following, EXCEPT:

A) hand gestures.

B) words.

C) facial expressions.

D) eye movement.

22. Which compensation is observed while performing the overhead squat at the lumbo/pelvic/hip complex when the individual is observed from the lateral view?

A) an asymmetrical weight shift in the hips

B) the low back rounding or arching

C) the arms falling forward

D) the knees adduct and internally rotate

23. A sarcomere is

   A) a myofibril.

   B) a type IIb muscle fiber.

   C) a site at which the motor neuron and muscle fibers are joined to form a chemical synapse.

   D) a contractile unit found in striated muscle that is connected end-to-end along myofibrils.

24. Examples of proprioceptors include

   A) Golgi tendon organs and slow-twitch muscle fibers.

   B) Golgi tendon organs and type I muscle fibers.

   C) muscle spindle fibers and Golgi tendon organs.

   D) muscle spindle fibers and striated muscle.

25. Length-tension relationships refer to

   A) the amount of actin-myosin crossbridges that occur within the sarcomeres, giving the muscle its range of motion.

   B) muscles working together to perform a particular body movement.

   C) muscles contracting in opposite directions to produce force around the same rotational axis.

   D) muscles contracting to move a joint beyond its typical range of motion.

26. The general cardio warm-up should start with what?

   A) dynamic stretching

   B) agility ladders

   C) cardiovascular training

   D) PNF stretching

27. _____together are considered the top tier of the allied healthcare continuum.

   A) Physicians and nurses

   B) Occupational and physical therapists

   C) Registered dieticians and certified nutritionists

   D) Personal trainers and health coaches

28. What is the most common order of periods throughout a program periodization?

   A) first transition period, preparatory period, competitive period, second transition period

   B) competitive period, first transition period, second transition period, preparatory period

   C) macrocycle, second transition period, competitive period, preparatory period

   D) preparatory period, first transition period, competitive period, second transition period

29. What are some physiological benefits of cooling down?

   A) promotes flexibility

   B) raises body temperature

   C) builds lean muscle mass

   D) mentally prepares a person for exercise

30. Which ergogenic aid is illegal in competition?

   A) carbohydrate loading

   B) blood doping

   C) vitamin supplements

   D) creatine

31. What is the primary compensation seen while observing the knees from the anterior view during the single-leg squat assessment?

   A) the hips hiking

   B) excessive rotation of the pelvis

   C) the knees moving inward toward the midline of the body

   D) the knees traveling over the toes

32. Choose the best answer that explains why the following is NOT a SMART goal:

   The client is starting her program in early April and would like to lose weight in the three months prior to her vacation at the end of June.

   A) The goal is not measurable.

   B) The goal is not action-oriented.

   C) The goal is not specific.

   D) The goal is not time-stamped.

33. Professionalism includes the following characteristics, EXCEPT:

   A) using profanity while speaking with their client.

   B) wearing proper and tasteful athletic attire.

   C) focusing only on the client.

   D) staying approachable by using open body language.

34. The pulmonary artery carries

   A) deoxygenated blood from the heart to the lungs.

   B) oxygenated blood from the lungs to the heart.

   C) oxygenated blood from the heart to the lungs.

   D) deoxygenated blood from the right atrium to the right ventricle.

35. Before beginning work with clients, what should the certified personal trainer acquire to help in emergency situations?

   A) personal liability insurance

   B) negligence insurance

   C) CPR, AED, and first aid certification

   D) a personal trainer certification

36. What happens to calcium ions during the relaxation phase of muscular contraction?

   A) They release the blockade of troponin and tropomyosin to allow for actin-myosin crossbridging.

   B) They return to the sarcoplasmic reticulum, allowing the blockade of troponin and tropomyosin to prevent crossbridging of actin and myosin.

   C) They are buffered by the muscle.

   D) Nothing happens to the calcium ions during the relaxation phase.

37. Which test would be the most appropriate for a prenatal client?

   A) overhead squat assessment

   B) one-repetition barbell squat

   C) 300-yard shuttle

   D) 1.5-mile run

38. What are the names of the food groups?

   A) vegetables, fruits, grains, protein, and dairy

   B) vegetables, fruits, grains, protein, dairy, and oils

   C) vegetables, fruits, grains, meat, and dairy

   D) vegetables, fruits, grains, sugar, and dairy

39. Undulating periodization is characterized by microcycles that follow

A) varying loads and volumes throughout a microcycle with increasing intensity over the course of the macrocycle.

B) one load and volume through an entire mesocycle.

C) a steady progression of load and volume through a mesocycle and gradual progression of intensity throughout the macrocycle.

D) no particular pattern in progressions of loading.

40. Which populations should not use SMR in their warm-up protocols?

A) a person with vitiligo

B) a person whose body fat exceeds 30 percent

C) a person who is prone to blood clots

D) a person who has no flexibility

41. DOMS stands for

A) Dynamic Onset Muscle Soreness.

B) Dynamic Onset Muscle Strength.

C) Delayed Onset Muscle Soreness.

D) Delayed Onset Muscle Strength.

42. Which method determines body fat by measuring body mass through the use of a highly precise scale while the individual sits inside the device?

A) DEXA scan

B) near-infrared interactance

C) bioelectrical impedance

D) air displacement plethysmography

43. The primary benefit of resistance training for muscles is to elicit the effect of muscle

A) hypertrophy.

B) atrophy.

C) hyperplasia.

D) fatigue.

44. What dictates the duration that a client should perform the SMR exercise?

A) the client's pain tolerance and sensitivity

B) the client's age

C) the client's fitness level

D) the client's flexibility

45. When designing an exercise program for clients focused on weight management, which training method may NOT be advisable for beginners due to excessive forces placed on the joints?

A) training for muscular power using plyometrics

B) training for muscular hypertrophy using resistance cable weights

C) training for muscular endurance using free weights

D) training for aerobic endurance using the recumbent bicycle

46. Negligence in training environments includes areas such as:

A) the client acting inappropriately.

B) an environmental emergency.

C) the client performing appropriately designed workouts with the trainer present.

D) equipment cleanliness.

47. Blood pressure is determined using

   A) an electrocardiogram.

   B) heart rate and ventilation rate.

   C) a sphygmomanometer.

   D) a pulse.

48. Orthostatic hypotension is commonly caused by

   A) height.

   B) training status.

   C) a change in blood pressure due to postural position.

   D) high blood pressure.

49. At what point should one hold a static stretch?

   A) as soon as feeling the stretch, before any discomfort

   B) at the point of intense pain

   C) at the point of slight discomfort

   D) The stretcher should pulse the stretch, not hold it.

50. Anyone interested in obtaining a personal training certification should make sure the certifying body is accredited by which organizations?

   A) HIPAA and the NCCA

   B) ANSI and NASM

   C) ACE and ACSM

   D) NCCA and ANSI

51. What is the primary purpose of the Balance Error Scoring System test?

   A) to assess single-leg strength

   B) to assess static postural stability

   C) to assess flexibility

   D) to assess strength and neuromuscular efficiency

52. Which exercise will benefit a football lineman MOST during the course of the game?

   A) bench press

   B) seated lateral pull-down

   C) standing military press

   D) push press

53. What is the energy expenditure for a 154 lb. man for one hour of jogging at 7 MET? (There is more than one correct answer.)

   A) 25 kcal

   B) 515 kcal

   C) 1132 kcal

   D) 490 kcal

54. Hyperventilation refers to

   A) increased breathing rate.

   B) increased blood pressure.

   C) increased sweating.

   D) decreased breathing rate.

55. What is the most challenging form of cardiorespiratory training?

   A) walking at an incline

   B) swimming with a kickboard

   C) using an elliptical machine

   D) jumping rope

56. What should the trainer make sure to do first, prior to starting a training program with a new client with medical concerns indicated on their medical history paperwork?

   A) set SMART goals

   B) make sure the client has been cleared by a physician for exercise

   C) perform a fitness assessment

   D) test the client's flexibility

57. A kinesthetic learner

   A) interprets information through watching the trainer do one or two reps while explaining.

   B) interprets information through listening to the trainer explain the movement.

   C) interprets information through a combination of watching the trainer while they explain where the client should feel the exercise.

   D) interprets the information through thinking through an explanation of the exercise.

58. While standing on the left leg during the Balance Error Scoring System test, which direction should be reached by the test subject's second attempt?

   A) lateral

   B) posterolateral

   C) anterior

   D) anteromedial

59. Over time, hypertension can lead to

   A) overuse injuries.

   B) musculoskeletal injuries.

   C) delayed onset muscle soreness.

   D) heart attacks and strokes.

60. The autonomic nervous system breaks down further into

   A) the peripheral nervous system and the central nervous system.

   B) the somatic nervous system and the parasympathetic nervous system.

   C) the parasympathetic nervous system and the sympathetic nervous system.

   D) the sympathetic nervous system and the central nervous system.

61. Where is the myelin sheath located?

   A) on the dendrites

   B) on the brain

   C) on the heart

   D) on the axons

62. What are the main electrolytes lost through sweating?

   A) calcium and magnesium

   B) chloride and phosphate

   C) sodium and chloride

   D) sodium and potassium

63. What can be considered a regression for the static straddle stretch?

   A) seated lean back

   B) butterfly stretch

   C) semi-straddle stretch

   D) supine knee stretch

64. A workout should always start with

   A) high-intensity exercises.

   B) flexibility training.

   C) small-muscle-group resistance training.

   D) a dynamic warm-up.

65. How are the BOD POD and underwater weighing similar?

   A) They can both be used in a fitness setting.

   B) They both compare volume to weight to determine body composition.

   C) They both can be directly correlated with BMI.

   D) They both involve water displacement.

66. When performing consecutive sets of an exercise, resistance training rest periods depend primarily upon the

A) load and volume.

B) strength of the client.

C) power of the client.

D) There is no rest period in resistance training.

67. Considering the differences between youth and adult clients, which assessment would be the LEAST beneficial for testing most youth clients?

A) one-repetition bench press test

B) push-up test

C) overhead squat assessment

D) sit-and-reach test

68. When would one use a dynamic stretch in the warm-up protocol?

A) as the first part of the warm-up protocol

B) before static stretching

C) only with advanced clients

D) as the last part of the warm-up protocol

69. Clients looking to improve strength gains will benefit most from

A) two days of resistance training and three days of cardiovascular training a week.

B) increasing resistance training to four days a week when using an upper body/lower body split program.

C) simply performing the same bodyweight workout two to three days a week.

D) training the same muscle groups on consecutive days, multiple times a week.

70. In the diagram below, which describes how to calculate a client's Q angle, how will a smaller pelvis influence the Q angle?

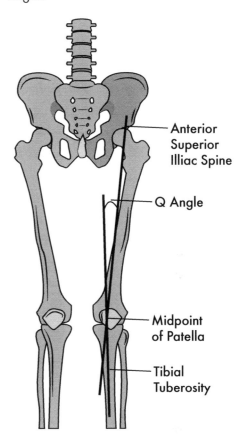

Anterior Superior Illiac Spine

Q Angle

Midpoint of Patella

Tibial Tuberosity

A) If the client has a small pelvis, then the Q angle will be small.

B) The size of a client's pelvis will not influence the Q angle.

C) If the client has a small pelvis, then the Q angle will be large.

D) Only a large pelvis will influence the Q angle.

71. A push press would be a progression for:

A) triceps extension

B) biceps barbell curl

C) step up

D) barbell shoulder press

72. Motor unit recruitment refers to

    A) the constant stimulus of a motor unit to produce a continuous contraction of muscle.

    B) the process of stimulating more motor units to overcome a force.

    C) the impulse sent for muscular contraction.

    D) type I muscle fibers.

73. What occurs at the end of the axon?

    A) a stimulus

    B) the sarcolemma

    C) actin and myosin

    D) the synapse

74. Which type of fluid is recommended during lengthy exercise?

    A) water

    B) sport drinks containing electrolytes and carbohydrates

    C) fruit juice

    D) caffeinated beverages

75. What is the purpose of the barbell squat assessment?

    A) to determine lower body muscular endurance

    B) to determine upper body strength

    C) to determine maximal lower body strength

    D) to determine single-leg strength

76. In general, as training volume goes down, training load

    A) goes up.

    B) goes down.

    C) stays the same.

    D) goes down for athletes only.

77. What type of dynamic stretch would be ideal for an upper body workout?

    A) arm swings

    B) lunge walk

    C) inverted hamstring

    D) walking over and under

78. In the power tier of resistance training, what should be the primary focus of an exercise regimen?

    A) fat loss

    B) force production

    C) proper form

    D) core strength

79. The power phase of training coincides with the _____ stage of learning.

    A) cognitive

    B) supportive

    C) autonomous

    D) associative

80. The endocrine system is made up of glands that

    A) secrete hormones for various functions.

    B) provide structural support for organs.

    C) produce forces for movement.

    D) have limited or no function.

81. When acquiring the required CECs, which of the following is NOT an acceptable option?

    A) workshops

    B) conferences

    C) exercise specialization certifications

    D) blog contributions

82. Testosterone is

   A) a gland.

   B) a catabolic hormone.

   C) an anabolic hormone.

   D) an organ.

83. What does the release of cortisol by the endocrine system stimulate?

   A) production of insulin

   B) production of melatonin

   C) production of epinephrine and norepinephrine

   D) production of parathyroid hormone

84. What is a good example of safe training practices?

   A) performing outdoor workouts regardless of weather conditions

   B) considering environmental factors prior to engaging in outdoor workouts

   C) using a parking lot for a workout

   D) relying on fitness center clientele to pick up equipment after usage

85. Which assessment predicts an individual's ability to repeatedly absorb the stress of continuous jumping?

   A) reactive strength index test

   B) vertical jump test

   C) Margaria-Kalamen test

   D) long jump test

86. What kind of training allows users to leverage their body weight to target muscle groups while working the core?

   A) plyometrics

   B) balance

   C) suspension

   D) cardiovascular

87. All the following aerobic machines use the upper body EXCEPT

   A) the recumbent bicycle.

   B) the rowing machine.

   C) the elliptical machine.

   D) the arm bicycle.

88. What volume and load are associated with the development of muscular hypertrophy?

   A) very light loads with very high volumes

   B) very heavy loads with very light volumes

   C) moderate volumes and loads

   D) very light volumes with light loads performed at a high velocity

89. Which exercise would likely induce the neuroendocrine response?

   A) biceps curls

   B) seated calf raises

   C) wrist extensions

   D) back squats

90. Time management is a _____ _____ tool.

   A) goal-setting

   B) relationship-building

   C) behavioral-change

   D) self-efficacy

91. Which types of goals does a personal trainer NOT address before beginning an exercise program?

   A) mental goals

   B) physical goals

   C) financial goals

   D) psychological goals

92. What are the muscular rings that allow for the movement of food through the digestive tract?

    A) the small intestine

    B) the rectum

    C) the stomach

    D) the sphincter

93. How does the pancreas affect those who are exercising?

    A) It regulates blood pressure.

    B) It regulates blood sugar.

    C) It regulates heart rate

    D) It regulates hydration status.

94. Which assessment would be most appropriate for athletes who want to improve their change-of-direction ability?

    A) the forty-yard dash

    B) the *t*-test

    C) the vertical jump test

    D) the hexagon test

95. Which of the following is NOT considered the proper standard for a personal trainer's business practices?

    A) Defend yourself with rude and slanderous remarks, should a disagreement arise with a peer or client.

    B) Comply with state regulations and guidelines for certified professionals.

    C) Be honest and tasteful with advertising.

    D) Maintain professional and supportive relationships with vendors and peers.

96. What is/are some very simple measurements that do NOT determine body fat percentage but can indicate whether a client is at a healthy weight?

    A) BMI, WHR, and waist circumference

    B) skinfold measurements, BMI, WHR, and waist circumference

    C) skinfold measurements

    D) skinfold measurements and BOD POD

97. When it comes to goal-setting strategies, what does the *S* in SMART stand for?

    A) start

    B) strong

    C) specific

    D) silly

98. What is the purpose of the 5-10-5 shuttle test?

    A) to assess lateral speed and agility

    B) to assess 180-degree direction-change ability, horizontal speed, and agility

    C) to assess the ability to run in the sagittal and frontal plane

    D) to assess an individual's maximal horizontal jumping distance

99. What does the sit-and-reach test assess?

    A) quadriceps flexibility

    B) shoulder flexibility

    C) lower back and hamstring flexibility

    D) hamstring strength

100. What type of movement is plyometrics?

    A) balance

    B) sprinting

    C) jumping

    D) sliding

101. What is a physiological benefit of resistance training?

A) increased flexibility

B) healthy skin

C) increased metabolism

D) longer stride

102. Cam machines are considered what type of machine?

A) hydraulic machine

B) cardiovascular machine

C) friction machine

D) air machine

103. What is a training plateau?

A) when the client has reached peak performance

B) when the trainer has the client performing the same workout on several consecutive training days

C) when the client is not seeing fitness improvements even though the client is still training

D) when the trainer progresses the client's program to reach a desired goal

104. The best anatomical structure to be described as a fulcrum in the human body is

A) a joint.

B) a bone.

C) a muscle.

D) an organ.

105. Scheduling negativity is a tool that helps combat

A) self-doubt.

B) positivity.

C) goal-setting.

D) exercise goals.

106. Which is the best example of a first-class lever in the human body?

A) the quadriceps muscle and knee

B) the biceps muscle and elbow

C) the muscles on the back of the neck and the skull on the first vertebrae

D) the muscles of the calf and the joint at the toes and ball of the foot

107. Which level in the training continuum should a client be in to implement plyometrics exercises in their routine?

A) Power

B) Strength

C) Stabilization

D) Core and Balance

108. When should a training program be progressed?

A) every workout

B) when the client has reached the cognitive phase of learning the exercises

C) when the client is still having significant delayed-onset muscle soreness

D) when the client has completed the workout without compensation in technique more than once

109. The medical history form is utilized to

A) protect trainers from liability if the client is injured.

B) assess potential medical concerns that may require a physician's clearance before the client can start an exercise program.

C) determine whether the client is interested in beginning an exercise program.

D) determine the intensity at which a client may begin an exercise program.

110. Which of the following methods represents the most effective way to lose weight and keep it off?

   A) reduce dietary intake by 400 kcal/day

   B) do weight bearing aerobic exercise for one hour every day

   C) reduce dietary intake by 1,000 kcal/day

   D) reduce caloric intake by 300 kcal/day and do a one-hour aerobic workout or jog four to five times per week

111. As time increases, the amount of force one can apply

   A) does not matter because the two components are unrelated.

   B) increases.

   C) stays the same.

   D) decreases.

112. Which of the following describes the amount of weight lifted in a single repetition, regardless of velocity?

   A) power

   B) force

   C) strength

   D) endurance

113. Which of the following is NOT a reason to reassess clients?

   A) to keep clients committed to the goals they have created

   B) to reevaluate goals

   C) to make sure the most appropriate exercises are being programmed to help the clients achieve their goals

   D) to introduce new assessments to see if the program is working

114. Fast feet and A-skips are ideal for

   A) speed, agility, and quickness warm-ups.

   B) agility cooldown.

   C) cardio endurance training.

   D) static stretches.

115. Steady-state cardiovascular activity is

   A) more intense than anaerobic endurance training.

   B) short-duration aerobic training of less than five minutes.

   C) good for power athletes like sprinters, football players, and Olympic lifters.

   D) appropriate for cross-country runners.

116. The anaerobic energy system requires

   A) oxygen for the creation of ATP molecules.

   B) creatine phosphate for the creation of ATP molecules.

   C) lactic acid for energy production.

   D) acetyl CoA for ATP production.

117. A client who smokes, is diagnosed as obese, and has a documented family history of heart attacks would be at what level of risk?

   A) no risk

   B) low risk

   C) intermediate risk

   D) high risk

118. What is a progression of a Romanian deadlift?

   A) push jerk

   B) upright row

   C) still-leg deadlift

   D) inverted hamstring

119. When conducting the three-minute step test, the metronome should be set to how many beats per minute?

    A) 96

    B) 108

    C) 24

    D) 48

120. Which cardiorespiratory fitness assessment would most accurately measure anaerobic capacity?

    A) a 1.5-mile run

    B) the 300-yard shuttle test

    C) the Rockport walk test

    D) the twelve-minute run test

121. Anabolism is

    A) the breakdown of molecules through metabolism.

    B) adenosine triphosphate.

    C) the building up of molecules through metabolism.

    D) the ability of the body to consume and use oxygen.

122. When training children, the fitness professional should focus primarily on

    A) increasing the amount of weight lifted.

    B) improving strength.

    C) improving technique and teaching proper form.

    D) improving power.

123. What type of exercise uses a free weight?

    A) hydraulic shoulder press

    B) air propelled rowing machine

    C) plyometric box jump

    D) dumbbell bench press

124. Professional growth doesn't just happen in a classroom or educational setting with textbooks and computer-based modules. A trainer can learn a lot from _____, _____, or _____, which allow the new trainer to shadow an experienced trainer while on the job.

    A) mentorships, ownerships, observations

    B) observations, internships, mentorships

    C) internships, leaderships, ownerships

    D) mentorships, internships, leaderships

125. Cone drills focus on

    A) speed training.

    B) quickness training.

    C) agility training.

    D) resistance training.

126. Performing cardiovascular exercise at near-maximal efforts (over 90 percent of maximum heart rate) will help to improve

    A) development of type I muscle fibers.

    B) recovery rate from a tough workout.

    C) lactate threshold and movement speed.

    D) decreased resting heart rate.

127. Athletes will generally have

    A) more coordination than untrained individuals.

    B) less strength when starting a fitness program.

    C) less coordination when starting a fitness program.

    D) more fatigue than untrained individuals.

128. What is the preferred pulse landmark for determining the resting heart rate?

A) carotid

B) femoral

C) brachial

D) radial

129. What does the systolic number represent?

A) pressure in the arterial system after the heart contracts

B) the point at which the pulse can no longer be felt

C) the pulse fading away

D) the sphygmomanometer

130. What exercise precaution should be taken when training a pregnant woman?

A) Training frequency should be reduced.

B) Resistance training should be eliminated.

C) Rest periods should be increased.

D) Abdominal exercises should be eliminated.

131. When is it acceptable to use a spotter?

A) The lifter has poor form and cannot lift the weight.

B) The lifter is using proper form but needs support to complete reps.

C) The lifter has poor form and can lift the weight.

D) The lifter wants a spotter.'

132. Which is NOT an example of a peptide hormone?

A) human growth hormone

B) testosterone

C) human chorionic gonadotropin

D) luteinizing hormone

133. The female athlete triad is made up of which three below?

A) amenorrhea, nutrition, and osteoporosis

B) amenorrhea, osteoporosis, and exercise

C) exercise, nutrition, and recovery

D) amenorrhea, disordered eating, and osteoporosis

134. Clients should complete the following forms, EXCEPT:

A) PAR-Q

B) medical disclosure

C) demographic form

D) client contract

135. The difference between the symptoms of DOMS and the symptoms of overtraining is

A) how sore the muscle is.

B) which muscles are sore.

C) nothing—DOMS is actually a symptom of overtraining.

D) whether the soreness is acute or chronic.

136. Which of the following is a sustainable way to lose weight and improve health?

A) supplementation with Garcinia cambogia

B) exercising in heavy or non-breathable clothing

C) a high-protein, high-fat, very low-carbohydrate diet

D) a moderately calorie-restricted, nutrient-rich, and varied diet coupled with regular exercise

137. All these muscle groups comprise the core EXCEPT

A) the hip adductor complex.

B) the erector spinae.

C) the biceps brachii.

D) the internal obliques.

138. What effect does age have on the cardiovascular system?

A) The cardiovascular system stays the same with age.

B) Maximal heart rate increases with age.

C) Maximal heart rate decreases with age.

D) The risk of atherosclerosis decreases with age.

139. What method is most commonly used by personal trainers to determine body fat?

A) skinfold measurements

B) body mass index

C) air displacement plethysmography

D) circumference measurements (to determine girth)

140. Clients with chronic obstructive pulmonary disease (COPD) have difficulty breathing and may require that their cardiovascular training

A) start at fifteen minutes per session, three days per week.

B) start at thirty minutes per session, three to five days per week.

C) start at thirty to sixty minutes per session, five days per week.

D) not start at all since COPD clients should not participate in cardiovascular exercise due to their difficulty in breathing.

141. Which of the following is NOT an aspect of anorexia?

A) a feeling of societal or sports-related pressure to maintain a very lean body

B) an insatiable desire for food

C) deficiencies of essential nutrients

D) extreme restriction of caloric intake

142. Even if a personal trainer is employed at a gym, he or she should invest in

A) his or her own fitness equipment.

B) liability insurance.

C) a computer.

D) business cards.

143. Due to an increased fall risk with older adults, what might the trainer include in an older adult's exercise program?

A) high intensity aerobic training

B) swimming

C) exercises to improve maximal strength in the upper body

D) exercises for improved balance during activities of daily living

144. Which disorder is defined by an insatiable desire to eat followed by extreme measures to compensate, such as purging or excessive exercise?

A) anorexia nervosa

B) obesity

C) bulimia nervosa

D) the female athlete triad

145. Which of the following assessments would precede a flexibility assessment?

A) physiological assessments

B) aerobic assessments

C) muscular endurance assessments

D) strength assessments

146. Which of the following is an example of a relative contraindication?

    A) recent history of myocardial infarction

    B) unstable angina

    C) uncontrolled symptomatic heart failure

    D) severe high blood pressure

147. Which of the following terms describes an individual's sense of his or her body position in space?

    A) muscle imbalance

    B) proprietary

    C) core control

    D) proprioception

148. The typical treatment for minor overtraining symptoms is to

    A) work the muscles at a lighter load.

    B) work the muscles at a lighter volume.

    C) temporarily stop exercising and get adequate rest.

    D) do cardiovascular exercise instead of resistance training.

149. To stay up-to-date with certification requirements, a personal trainer should do all of the following EXCEPT

    A) keep up-to-date with current health and fitness research.

    B) remain in good standing with a current certifying agency by obtaining necessary continuing education.

    C) arrive at training sessions at least ten minutes early.

    D) hold a valid certification in Cardiopulmonary Resuscitation (CPR)/Automated External Defibrillator (AED).

150. Which acronym is used in determining whether someone is having a stroke?

    A) DOMS

    B) FAST

    C) EPOC

    D) RICE

1. A) Incorrect. *Organ systems* are larger than *organs*.

B) Correct. This answer correctly lists the structures from largest to smallest.

C) Incorrect. The *organ system* is smaller than *organism,* and *tissue* is smaller than *organ.*

D) Incorrect. This is the biological hierarchy from smallest to largest.

2. A) Incorrect. The heart is larger than just a cell.

B) Incorrect. The heart is larger than just a tissue.

C) Incorrect. The heart is a smaller part of an organ system.

D) Correct. The heart is an organ.

3. A) Incorrect. One should still be inhaling at this point.

B) Correct. Exhaling on exertion will help control and propel the user's force to complete the full range of motion.

C) Incorrect. The user should inhale through the stretch of the exercise allowing for the breath and potential energy to be ready for the contraction of the muscle.

D) Incorrect. This is not a part of muscle contraction.

4. A) Incorrect. The extent to which test scores correspond with future performance is predictive validity.

B) Incorrect. The measure of the degree of consistency or repeatability of a test is reliability.

C) Correct. Criterion referenced validity is the extent to which test scores are related to an outcome with another test of the same ability.

D) Incorrect. Validity is the degree to which a test measures what it is supposed to measure.

5. A) Incorrect. These are six steps in effective goal-setting, according to

the National Association of Sports Medicine (NASM).

B) Incorrect. These are six tools or techniques in behavior change.

C) Correct. These are the six phases of the readiness-to-change model.

D) Incorrect. Five of these words are the five tiers of the social-ecological behavior model. The sixth word, introvert, is a personality type.

6. A) Incorrect. The ability to distinguish between two different concepts is discriminant validity.

B) Incorrect. Test scores that must correspond with future performance demonstrate predictive validity.

C) Incorrect. The face validity of a test measures what the test has been designed to measure.

D) Correct. A test is said to be reliable if it delivers the same score or result.

7. A) Incorrect. The shoulders are observed as neither elevated nor rounded from the anterior view.

B) Incorrect. The knees are observed as neither flexed nor extended from the lateral view.

C) Correct. The shoulders should maintain a normal kyphotic curve and not be excessively rounded when viewed from the lateral angle.

D) Incorrect. The head should be observed as neither tilted nor rotated while observing from the anterior view.

8. **A) Correct.** Kyphosis is excessive posterior curvature of the spine, while lordosis is anterior.

B) Incorrect. Kyphosis and lordosis have opposite meanings of what is expressed in the question.

C) Incorrect. Lateral curvature refers to scoliosis.

D) Incorrect. The two terms have opposite meanings and are not interchangeable.

9. A) Incorrect. Biaxial joints only allow for freedom of movement in two planes of motion.

    B) Incorrect. Hinge joints typically only allow for freedom of movement in one plane of motion.

    C) Incorrect. A saddle joint has range of motion through multiple planes of motion; however, they do not allow for rotation around an axis.

    D) Correct. Ball-and-socket joints allow for the most freedom of movement.

10. A) Incorrect. Carbohydrates provide 4 kcal/gram; this is less than fat.

    B) Incorrect. Sugars are a type of carbohydrate and provide 4 kcal/gram.

    C) Correct. Fats provide 9 kcal/gram; this is more than carbohydrates or protein.

    D) Incorrect. Protein, like carbohydrates, provides 4 kcal/gram.

11. A) Incorrect. The gradual increase in intensity throughout an exercise program refers to *progression*.

    B) Correct. Regression is the reduction or modification of an exercise due to physical limitation or poor technique.

    C) Incorrect. Performing an exercise through one full range of motion is a *repetition*.

    D) Incorrect. The downward movement phase during the repetition of an exercise is the *eccentric phase*.

12. A) Incorrect. The ACSM provides personal training certifications; however, it does not provide CPR, AED, or first-aid certifications.

    B) Incorrect. Though courses may be held at local hospitals, the leading organizations that provide this training are the American Heart Association, OSHA, and the Red Cross.

    C) Incorrect. Personal trainer insurance organizations do not provide CPR, AED, or first-aid training.

    D) Correct. The AHA, OSHA, and the Red Cross are reliable organizations for obtaining certifications in CPR, AED, and first aid.

13. A) Incorrect. The personal trainer's response must be to refer the client to a certified nutritionist or registered dietitian.

    B) Incorrect. Even if the trainer has direct knowledge of the product, unless certified in its use, he cannot discuss nutrition supplements with a client.

    C) Incorrect. Regardless of his personal experience with a dietary supplement, a trainer must not discuss supplements with a client unless the trainer has an additional nutrition certification.

    D) Correct. The personal trainer can respond only if he has a nutrition certification that expands his scope of practice.

14. A) Incorrect. Bone mineral density develops more easily during childhood.

    B) Correct. Bone mineral density develops more easily during childhood.

    C) Incorrect. Though exercise does help to improve bone density later in life, it is developed more easily during childhood.

    D) Incorrect. Bone mineral density declines and the potential for osteoporosis increases in the elderly.

15. A) Incorrect. Power muscles are considered Type II muscle groups. They are larger and tire easily.

    B) Incorrect. Weak muscles are not a type of muscle group.

    C) Correct. Postural muscles, or core muscles, are slow to fatigue, which are Type I muscles.

    D) Incorrect. Leg muscles fall into the Type II muscle group.

16. A) Incorrect. The weight lifted for a single repetition is the *load*.

    B) Incorrect. Performing a specific number of repetitions through their full range refers to a *set*.

C) Incorrect. The principle of gradually increasing difficulty to elicit muscular adaptation through the course of the periodization is the *overload principle*.

D) **Correct.** Volume is the number of sets multiplied by the number of repetitions of an exercise.

17. **A)** **Correct.** Signage should be placed in a visible location on the equipment, indicating that the equipment is malfunctioning and should not be used.

B) Incorrect. Clients may not realize which piece of equipment the trainer is talking about and could injure themselves if they mistakenly use it.

C) Incorrect. Clients may be injured by broken equipment, so signage indicating the equipment is out of order should always be placed on the equipment immediately, before a client might inadvertently use it.

D) Incorrect. Certain pieces of equipment may have warranties and may require a technician's support. The fitness professional should not disassemble equipment.

18. A) Incorrect. The fat-soluble vitamins have no direct role in energy metabolism.

B) Incorrect. Antioxidants neutralize free radicals which can be a side effect of energy metabolism, but they are not directly involved in energy metabolism.

C) **Correct.** All of the B vitamins—except folate and B-12—are involved in energy metabolism.

D) Incorrect. Folate and B-12 are involved in transferring single carbons and deficiencies in intake manifest mainly as megaloblastic anemia.

19. A) Incorrect. This view only examines three of the five kinetic chain checkpoints.

B) Incorrect. This view only examines two of the five kinetic chain checkpoints.

C) **Correct.** Each kinetic chain checkpoint should be viewed during the static postural assessment.

D) Incorrect. This view only examines two of the five kinetic chain checkpoints.

20. A) Incorrect. This is what is affected by osteoporosis.

B) Incorrect. Lordosis is excessive anterior curvature of the lumbar spine.

C) Incorrect. Scoliosis is excessive lateral curvature of the spine.

D) **Correct.** Osteopenia is the precursor to osteoporosis.

21. A) Incorrect. Hand gestures are body language.

B) **Correct.** Words are verbal communication.

C) Incorrect. Facial expressions are body language.

D) Incorrect. Eye movement is body language.

22. A) Incorrect. An asymmetrical weight shift in the hips would be seen from the posterior view.

B) **Correct.** The lower back rounding or arching would be seen from the lateral view.

C) Incorrect. The arms falling forward would be observed at the shoulder joint.

D) Incorrect. The knees adducting and internally rotating would be observed at the knee joint.

23. A) Incorrect. Myofibrils contain sarcomeres.

B) Incorrect. This is a type of fast-twitch muscle fiber.

C) Incorrect. This is the neuromuscular junction.

D) **Correct.** This is the definition of a sarcomere.

24. A) Incorrect. Slow-twitch muscle fibers are not proprioceptors.

B) Incorrect. Type I muscle fibers are not proprioceptors.

C) **Correct.** These are two examples of proprioceptors.

D) Incorrect. Striated muscle is not a proprioceptor.

25. **A)** **Correct.** This is the definition of a length-tension relationship in muscle.

B) Incorrect. This refers to muscular synergists.

C) Incorrect. This refers to force-couple relationships.

D) Incorrect. This refers to hyperextension.

26. A) Incorrect. Warm-ups should start with general conditioning and end with dynamic stretches.

B) Incorrect. Agility training is too high of intensity.

C) **Correct.** This training can be modified for any fitness level and provides a general conditioning allowing the body temp to rise.

D) Incorrect. PNF stretching should not be done with cold muscles.

27. **A)** **Correct.** Physicians and nurses are considered the top tier of the continuum.

B) Incorrect. Occupational and physical therapists are not the top tier of the continuum.

C) Incorrect. Registered dieticians and certified nutritionists are not the top tier of the continuum.

D) Incorrect. Personal trainers and health coaches are not the top tier of the continuum.

28. A) Incorrect. The sequence is out of order.

B) Incorrect. The sequence is out of order.

C) Incorrect. A macrocycle contains all of the periods.

D) **Correct.** This is the most common order of periods.

29. **A)** **Correct.** Stretching should be part of a cooldown routine, since the muscles have been worked and are still warm.

B) Incorrect. This is a benefit of warming up the body before exercising.

C) Incorrect. This is a benefit of resistance training.

D) Incorrect. This is another benefit of warm-ups.

30. A) Incorrect. Carbohydrate loading is legal and simply involves a specific dietary regimen prior to competition.

B) **Correct.** Blood doping is illegal as it gives an unnatural advantage and can also be dangerous.

C) Incorrect. Vitamin supplements are just normal nutrients in supplement form and are legal.

D) Incorrect. Creatine is a normal component of food and can be taken legally in supplement form.

31. A) Incorrect. The hips hiking is a compensation seen at the lumbo/pelvic/hip complex.

B) Incorrect. Excessive rotation of the pelvis is observed at the lumbo/pelvic/hip complex.

C) **Correct.** The knees moving inward toward the midline of the body is the primary compensation seen at the knee checkpoint during the single-leg squat assessment.

D) Incorrect. The knees traveling over the toes is not the primary compensation seen at the knee during the single-leg squat assessment.

32. A) Incorrect. The goal is measurable because the trainer is able to weigh the client on a scale.

B) Incorrect. The goal is action-oriented because it requires the client to actively participate in the fitness program to achieve the goal.

C) **Correct.** The goal is not specific. The client neglected to decide how much weight to lose prior to her vacation.

D) Incorrect. The goal is time-stamped because the client wants to complete it prior to the vacation start date.

33. **A)** **Correct.** A trainer should refrain from the use of profanity while speaking with a client.

B) Incorrect. Trainers should always look the part; avoid jeans or clothing that is revealing or too tight.

C) Incorrect. A trainer should always be attentive to the client, especially in a session. Avoid talking on cell phones or texting.

D) Incorrect. Personal trainers should always be approachable and available to answer any questions.

34. **A)** **Correct.** The pulmonary artery is the artery that transports blood from the heart to the lungs for oxygen collection.

B) Incorrect. This refers to the pulmonary vein.

C) Incorrect. This pathway does not make sense as the blood is already oxygenated.

D) Incorrect. There is no artery carrying blood from heart chamber to heart chamber.

35. A) Incorrect. Although it's a good idea to have personal liability insurance for legal protection, it will not help trainers in emergency situations.

B) Incorrect. Negligence insurance should be included in adequate personal trainer liability insurance.

C) **Correct.** CPR, AED, and first aid certifications qualify the trainer to be a first responder in emergency situations; these certifications should be obtained prior to the trainer beginning work with clients.

D) Incorrect. Although a personal trainer certification helps to improve expertise in fitness, the certification does not include emergency responder training.

36. A) Incorrect. This occurs during the contraction phase.

B) **Correct.** The calcium returns to the sarcoplasmic reticulum, and crossbridging is again prevented.

C) Incorrect. Buffering does not occur.

D) Incorrect. Calcium ions play an important role throughout the process.

37. **A)** **Correct.** The overhead squat would be the most appropriate exercise test for a prenatal client.

B) Incorrect. The intensity of the one-repetition barbell squat test would not be appropriate for a prenatal client

due to the high load and spinal loading of the barbell.

C) Incorrect. The intensity of the 300-yard shuttle test would not be appropriate for a prenatal client.

D) Incorrect. The 1.5-mile run test would not be the best option for a prenatal client; the Rockport walk test would be more appropriate due to its low intensity and shorter duration.

38. **A)** **Correct.** These are the five food groups designated by the Food Pyramid Guide and MyPlate program.

B) Incorrect. Oils are not considered a food group and should be used sparingly.

C) Incorrect. The more general term *protein* is used to refer to high-protein foods, examples of which are meat and seafood.

D) Incorrect. Sugar is not considered a food group and should be consumed sparingly.

39. **A)** **Correct.** The load and volume of an undulating program vary within a microcycle and progress steadily over the course of the periodization.

B) Incorrect. This pattern describes no particular progression or periodization.

C) Incorrect. This pattern describes a *linear periodization* rather than undulating.

D) Incorrect. There is no periodization that follows this pattern.

40. A) Incorrect. Vitiligo is a non-contagious skin condition.

B) Incorrect. Obesity is not a restricted special population for SMR.

C) **Correct.** Blood clots can move from the roller's pressure, causing an increased risk for them to travel to the heart, so SMR would not be recommended.

D) Incorrect. SMR would help a person who is inflexible release tension from strained muscle fibers.

41. A) Incorrect. The use of the word *dynamic* is not correct.

B) Incorrect. The use of the words *dynamic* and *strength* are not correct.

C) **Correct.** DOMS stands for Delayed Onset Muscle Soreness.

D) Incorrect. The use of the word *strength* is not correct.

42. A) Incorrect. The DEXA scan uses two x-ray beams to measure bone density levels.

B) Incorrect. Near-infrared interactance uses probes that emit infrared light that passes through muscle and fat.

C) Incorrect. Bioelectrical impedance uses a low-level electrical signal to help estimate body fat percentage.

D) **Correct.** Air displacement plethysmography uses a highly precise scale to help determine body fat percentage.

43. A) **Correct.** Resistance training elicits muscular hypertrophy and, subsequently, increased strength.

B) Incorrect. Resistance training prevents muscular atrophy.

C) Incorrect. Although hyperplasia may be a benefit, it is not well understood as the primary benefit of resistance training.

D) Incorrect. Muscular fatigue does occur as a result of resistance training, but it is not the primary benefit.

44. A) **Correct.** SMR can be uncomfortable, so the client should perform the exercise as long they can tolerate; between 30 – 60 seconds.

B) Incorrect. Age is not a factor.

C) Incorrect. Clients of any fitness level can use SMR.

D) Incorrect. Being flexible is not a factor.

45. A) **Correct.** Due to excessive forces placed on the joints by plyometric exercises, beginner programs may not require muscular power exercises.

B) Incorrect. Training for muscular hypertrophy is beneficial to clients looking to lose weight because it helps to change their body composition by increasing muscle mass and increasing resting metabolism.

C) Incorrect. Training for muscular endurance helps build a foundation to prevent muscular fatigue and promote neuromotor control.

D) Incorrect. Training for aerobic endurance is beneficial for clients focusing on weight management because it helps improve body composition by utilizing the body's adipose tissue as a fuel source.

46. A) Incorrect. Clients acting inappropriately is not negligence on the part of the trainer; however, the trainer should attempt to limit this behavior.

B) Incorrect. Environmental emergencies are not due to negligence.

C) Incorrect. The client performing appropriately designed workouts with the trainer present reduces the risk of negligence.

D) **Correct.** Equipment that is not cleaned regularly can lead to the spread of infectious diseases, resulting in a negligence lawsuit.

47. A) Incorrect. This device is used for measuring the heart's electrical signal.

B) Incorrect. Blood pressure cannot be determined this way.

C) **Correct.** The device to determine blood pressure is a sphygmomanometer.

D) Incorrect. This is used to determine heart rate.

48. A) Incorrect. Height is not the common cause of orthostatic hypotension.

B) Incorrect. Training status does not cause orthostatic hypotension.

C) **Correct.** Orthostatic hypotension is caused by a change in blood pressure due to postural position.

D) Incorrect. High blood pressure is not the common cause for orthostatic hypotension.

49. A) Incorrect. The intention of static stretching is to challenge the fibers.

    B) Incorrect. While it is important to seek a challenge, stretching should never be intensely painful; the individual risks pulling the muscle.

    C) **Correct.** Slight discomfort alerts the stretcher that he is challenging his range of motion, but allows him to hold the stretch.

    D) Incorrect. Stretchers should never bounce in a stretch; they could unintentionally pull a muscle.

50. A) Incorrect. This is only half correct; NCCA is an accreditation organization, but HIPAA is a patient health confidentiality act.

    B) Incorrect. This is only half correct; NASM is a certifying body and not an accreditation organization.

    C) Incorrect. ACE and ACSM are both certifying organizations, not accreditation organizations.

    D) **Correct.** NCCA and ANSI are the accreditation organizations that hold certifying bodies to a certain educational standard.

51. A) Incorrect. Static single-leg strength can be assessed, but it is not the primary purpose of the BESS assessment.

    B) **Correct.** The primary objective of the BESS test is to assess an individual's static postural stability.

    C) Incorrect. The flexibility of the standing leg is not being assessed.

    D) Incorrect. Assessing strength and neuromuscular efficiency is not the primary objective of the BESS test.

52. A) Incorrect. The bench press does not involve the core or leg muscles that are necessary for a football lineman's position.

    B) Incorrect. The seated lateral pull-down also eliminates use of the legs and is not specific to the position.

    C) Incorrect. Although the standing military press may benefit the player, since it includes the core and leg muscles, it is not the MOST beneficial exercise on the list because it does not develop power.

    D) **Correct.** The push-press forces athletes to generate power using their legs, stabilize with their core, and transmit force from the legs through the arms in a pushing motion. These are all specific to the common movements associated with a football lineman.

53. A) Incorrect. This is the product of MET × 3.5. There are more terms to the calculation.

    B) **Correct.** The formula: 7 MET × 3.5 mL oxygen/kg/minute × 70 kg × 60 minutes × 1 L/1000 mL × 5 kcal/L = 515 kcal provides an accurate energy expenditure for the person described in the question.

    C) Incorrect. Body weight must be converted from pounds to kilograms.

    D) **Correct.** The formula: 7 MET × 1 kcal/kg/hour × 70 kg × 1 hour = 490 kcal provides an accurate energy expenditure for the person described in the question. (Note: this answer is close to answer choice B, which is also correct. So, approximately 500 kcal will be burned by a 154 lb. man who jogs for one hour at 7 MET.)

54. **A)** **Correct.** This is the definition of hyperventilation.

    B) Incorrect. This is hypertension.

    C) Incorrect. This is a common reaction to increased exercise intensity.

    D) Incorrect. This is hypoventilation.

55. A) Incorrect. While walking at an incline is challenging, it does not use the full body.

    B) Incorrect. Swimming with a kickboard is challenging, but it does not use the arms and is low impact.

C) Incorrect. While an elliptical machine challenges both the upper and lower body, it is less intense than jumping rope.

D) Correct. Jumping rope requires the user to recruit their full body and it is higher impact than the other choices.

56. A) Incorrect. Setting SMART goals should be done prior to program design, but the client has medical concerns that need to be addressed.

B) Correct. If the client has a medical concern that may be affected by exercise, the client should see a physician to make sure she is healthy enough to begin an exercise program.

C) Incorrect. The fitness assessment may exacerbate a medical concern such as heart arrhythmias, high blood pressure, etc.

D) Incorrect. Flexibility tests are typically included in the fitness assessment and can create problems for clients with existing medical conditions.

57. A) Incorrect. This is a description of a visual learner.

B) Incorrect. This is a description of an auditory learner.

C) Correct. This is a description of a kinesthetic learner.

D) Incorrect. This does not describe visual, auditory, or kinesthetic learning.

58. A) Incorrect. A lateral reach is performed on the seventh reach.

B) Incorrect. A posterolateral reach is performed on the sixth reach.

C) Incorrect. To initiate the test, an anterior reach is performed on the first reach.

D) Correct. An anteromedial reach is performed on the second reach attempt.

59. A) Incorrect. Hypertension leads to cardiovascular events and is not typically related to overuse injuries.

B) Incorrect. Musculoskeletal injuries are typically related to overtraining or physical trauma.

C) Incorrect. Delayed onset muscle soreness, or DOMS, is the natural physiological result of overloading the muscle and is a normal occurrence.

D) Correct. Hypertension can lead to heart attacks and strokes.

60. A) Incorrect. These are the larger hierarchical nervous systems.

B) Incorrect. The somatic nervous system is incorrect.

C) Correct. These are the two branches of the autonomic nervous system.

D) Incorrect. The central nervous system is incorrect.

61. A) Incorrect. It is not found on the dendrites.

B) Incorrect. It is not found on the brain.

C) Incorrect. It is not found on the heart.

D) Correct. It is found on the axons.

62. A) Incorrect. Calcium and magnesium are lost in only small amounts in sweat.

B) Incorrect. Chloride and phosphate are lost in only small amounts in sweat.

C) Incorrect. Sweat results in a significant loss of sodium but not in chloride.

D) Correct. While all of these ions can be lost in sweat, sodium and potassium are the electrolytes that experience the most significant losses.

63. A) Incorrect. The seated lean back is a stretch for the shoulders, not the adductors.

B) Incorrect. The butterfly stretch is an adductor-only stretch; the straddle stretches the hamstrings and adductors.

C) Correct. The semi-straddle stretch allows one adductor and hamstring to be stretched at a time.

D) Incorrect. The supine knee stretch is a stretch for the hamstring and hip flexor.

64. A) Incorrect. This is dangerous because the muscles are not prepared for exercise yet.

B) Incorrect. Flexibility training involving static stretching and PNF stretching should be saved for last.

C) Incorrect. This is dangerous since the muscles are not prepared for exercise yet.

D) Correct. A dynamic warm-up that addresses the muscles that will be utilized during the workout should be done first.

65. A) Incorrect. Underwater weighing is generally only available in a research setting.

B) Correct. Both measure volume by measuring the displacement of water or air and compare it to weight to determine the percentage of body fat.

C) Incorrect. BMI is a measurement of weight versus height and does not give complete information about body composition as does a measurement of weight versus volume.

D) Incorrect. The BOD POD involves air displacement.

66. **A) Correct.** The load and volume of an exercise will primarily determine the rest period in between consecutive sets of that exercise.

B) Incorrect. The strength of the client will help to determine the weight rather than the rest period.

C) Incorrect. The power of the client determines the velocity at which an exercise is performed.

D) Incorrect. The rest period allows for adequate recovery of muscle energy systems to perform the exercise at the same load properly.

67. **A) Correct.** The one-repetition bench press test would be the least beneficial for testing most youth clients.

B) Incorrect. The push-up up test would be a beneficial assessment for testing the muscular strength and muscular endurance of youth clients.

C) Incorrect. The overhead squat would be a beneficial assessment for youth clients to help determine dynamic

movement efficiency and dynamic flexibility.

D) Incorrect. The sit-and-reach test would be beneficial to assess lower back and hamstring flexibility.

68. A) Incorrect. A dynamic stretch is the last part of the warm-up.

B) Incorrect. Dynamic stretches come after static stretching.

C) Incorrect. A dynamic stretch is appropriate for all fitness levels.

D) Correct. A dynamic stretch is the last part of the warm-up. These stretches more intensely target the muscle groups used in the exercise routine than the general cardio warm-up does.

69. A) Incorrect. Though this is beneficial for general health benefits, clients looking to increase strength will benefit more from increasing the resistance training frequency to more than two days a week.

B) Correct. A four-day split routine will provide adequate stimulation for improved strength.

C) Incorrect. Performing the same bodyweight workout two to three days a week will eventually become too easy and not provoke an overload effect.

D) Incorrect. Training the same muscle groups on consecutive days, multiple times a week may cause overtraining and potential injury.

70. **A) Correct.** A small pelvis will typically create a small Q angle, as typically seen in males.

B) Incorrect. The size of the pelvis can affect the size of the Q angle.

C) Incorrect. A small pelvis will not typically create a large Q angle.

D) Incorrect. The size of the pelvis will influence the Q angle no matter how large or small.

71. A) Incorrect. The primary mover for the triceps extension is the triceps; the

exercise does not share a similar movement pattern with the push press.

B) Incorrect. The primary mover for the biceps barbell curl is the biceps; the exercise does not share a similar movement pattern with the push press.

C) Incorrect. The primary mover for the step up is the lower body; the exercise does not share a similar movement pattern with the push press.

D) Correct. The barbell shoulder press is the same move as the push press, except it does not require a shallow squat to initiate a forced repetition. The primary movers are the shoulders, as in the push press.

72. A) Incorrect. This refers to summation.

B) Correct. This is the definition of motor unit recruitment.

C) Incorrect. This is nerve transmission to muscle.

D) Incorrect. This is a type of muscle fiber.

73. A) Incorrect. This is what creates an impulse.

B) Incorrect. This is found in the muscle fiber.

C) Incorrect. This is found at the level of the sarcomere.

D) Correct. The synapse occurs at the end of an axon.

74. A) Incorrect. While water can be used for short-term hydration, it can also dilute electrolytes during lengthy exercise. It is necessary to replace lost electrolytes.

B) Correct. Sport drinks replace both fluid and electrolytes and have the added advantage of supplying blood glucose for fuel.

C) Incorrect. While fruit juice does contain some electrolytes and carbohydrates, the sugars are too concentrated, resulting in slow gastric emptying and fluid absorption.

D) Incorrect. While a caffeinated beverage an hour prior to exercise might have benefits, caffeine is a diuretic and could decrease hydration

during exercise. For proper hydration during exercise, it is best to replace fluid and electrolytes and provide glucose for fuel.

75. A) Incorrect. The barbell squat assessment is used to test maximal strength, not muscular endurance.

B) Incorrect. The barbell squat assessment is used to determine lower body strength, not upper body strength.

C) Correct. The barbell squat assessment is used to test an individual's maximal lower body strength.

D) Incorrect. The barbell squat assessment is used to determine bilateral strength, not unilateral strength.

76. **A) Correct.** As training volume goes down, the load lifted should increase.

B) Incorrect. This is the opposite of what should happen.

C) Incorrect. Without increasing the load, decreasing the volume may cause a loss of overload, leading to lack of progression.

D) Incorrect. All clients will benefit from increasing the load while decreasing the volume.

77. **A) Correct.** Arm swings target the chest, back, shoulders, and arms.

B) Incorrect. Lunge walks are lower-body intensive.

C) Incorrect. The inverted hamstring stretch targets the lower body and core.

D) Incorrect. Walking over and under targets the lower body and primes the legs for lateral movement.

78. A) Incorrect. This is a prime focus of stabilization training.

B) Correct. Increasing force production in prime movers is the focus of power training.

C) Incorrect. Feedback on proper form is more of a focus in stability training, even though form is always a factor in strength training.

D) Incorrect. Building core strength is mostly focused on in stabilization training.

79. A) Incorrect. This stage of learning coincides with the stabilization training phase.

    B) Incorrect. This is a form of feedback, not learning.

    C) Correct. At this stage of learning, the movement is almost second nature to the client.

    D) Incorrect. This stage of learning coincides with the Strength Training Phase.

80. **A) Correct.** The glands of the endocrine system secrete hormones for various bodily functions.

    B) Incorrect. The muscles and connective tissues support the organs.

    C) Incorrect. The muscles produce forces for movement.

    D) Incorrect. The glands have many various functions.

81. A) Incorrect. Workshops are among the acceptable options to gain CECs.

    B) Incorrect. Conferences are acceptable ways to gain CECs.

    C) Incorrect. Among the acceptable CEC options are exercise specialization certifications.

    D) Correct. Blog contributions are not an acceptable way to acquire CECs.

82. A) Incorrect. Testosterone is a hormone secreted by a gland.

    B) Incorrect. Testosterone is an anabolic hormone.

    C) Correct. Testosterone is an anabolic hormone.

    D) Incorrect. Testosterone is not an organ.

83. A) Incorrect. The pancreas is responsible for insulin production.

    B) Incorrect. The pineal gland is responsible for melatonin production.

C) **Correct.** Cortisol release stimulates the production of epinephrine and norepinephrine.

D) Incorrect. The parathyroid is responsible for parathyroid hormone production.

84. A) Incorrect. Weather conditions directly impact client safety because they can lead to slip-and-fall injuries.

    B) Correct. When engaging in outdoor workouts, the fitness professional should consider environmental factors, such as heat, cold, rain, snow, ice, fallen leaves, etc.

    C) Incorrect. Prior to engaging in the workout, the fitness professional needs to determine all potentially hazardous conditions, such as gravel, traffic, fallen leaves, and other environmental factors.

    D) Incorrect. Though fitness professionals should encourage all clients to clean up their equipment following a workout, to ensure safety, the trainer should be responsible for this task.

85. **A) Correct.** The reactive strength index test is used to determine an individual's plyometric capacity by measuring jump reactive ability.

    B) Incorrect. The vertical jump test measures an individual's maximum vertical jump height.

    C) Incorrect. The Margaria-Kalamen test measures lower body power.

    D) Incorrect. The long jump test measures an individual's maximal horizontal jumping distance.

86. A) Incorrect. Plyometrics uses explosive movements to target muscle groups and core.

    B) Incorrect. Balance increases proprioception while building core strength.

    C) Correct. Suspension training allows the user to leverage his or her own body weight at different angles to target muscle groups while using the core as well.

D) Incorrect. Load-bearing activities are not considered cardiovascular training.

87. **A)** **Correct.** The recumbent bicycle is a leg powered machine.

B) Incorrect. The rowing machine uses the upper and lower body.

C) Incorrect. The elliptical machine uses the upper and lower body.

D) Incorrect. The arm bicycle uses the upper body only.

88. A) Incorrect. This load and volume range is associated with muscular endurance development.

B) Incorrect. This load and volume is associated with muscular strength gains.

C) **Correct.** Muscular hypertrophy involves performing moderate volumes of moderate loads.

D) Incorrect. Since velocity is the goal, these volumes and loads are for power development.

89. A) Incorrect. This exercise works smaller muscle groups and likely will not influence the neuroendocrine response.

B) Incorrect. This exercise works smaller muscle groups and likely will not influence the neuroendocrine response.

C) Incorrect. This exercise works smaller muscle groups and likely will not influence the neuroendocrine response.

D) **Correct.** Back squats work large muscle groups throughout the body and will likely stimulate the neuroendocrine response to exercise.

90. A) Incorrect. Time management is not a tool for setting goals.

B) Incorrect. Time management is not a tool for building relationships.

C) **Correct.** Time management is a tool for changing behaviors.

D) Incorrect. Time management is not a tool to build self-efficacy.

91. A) Incorrect. Personal trainers will help their clients set mental goals. Mental goals may allow clients to overcome mental barriers that could interfere with accomplishing their overall goals.

B) Incorrect. Personal trainers will help their clients set physical goals. Most clients will want to change their physical appearance when they begin working with a personal trainer.

C) **Correct.** Personal trainers will not help their clients set financial goals as these are out of their scope of practice.

D) Incorrect. Personal trainers will help their clients set psychological goals. Psychological goals may be determined in an effort to use exercise to combat common psychological problems, such as anxiety and stress.

92. A) Incorrect. This is a tube-like structure for nutrient absorption.

B) Incorrect. This is for the storage of feces before waste excretion.

C) Incorrect. This is for the breakdown of food using acidic liquid.

D) **Correct.** Sphincters are found throughout the digestive tract and are muscular rings that regulate food movement.

93. A) Incorrect. It does not regulate blood pressure.

B) **Correct.** It secretes insulin for blood sugar regulation.

C) Incorrect. It does not regulate heart rate.

D) Incorrect. It does not regulate hydration status.

94. A) Incorrect. The forty-yard dash is used to measure straight-ahead speed.

B) Incorrect. The *t*-test assesses an individual's ability to move forward, backward, and laterally but may not be the most accurate test for change-of-direction ability.

C) Incorrect. The vertical jump test is used to assess an individual's maximal vertical jump height.

D) **Correct.** The hexagon test is used to determine an individual's ability to change directions at a high speed.

95. **A)** **Correct.** Making rude and slanderous remarks is NOT the proper way for a personal trainer to handle a disagreement.

B) Incorrect. Complying with state regulations and guidelines is a fundamental part of a trainer's business practices.

C) Incorrect. Honest and tasteful advertising is to be expected in a trainer's business practices.

D) Incorrect. Maintaining professional and supportive relationships with vendors and peers is a standard part of a trainer's business practices.

96. **A)** **Correct.** These are very simple measurements that can be made with a tape measure and scale, and although they are not directly relatable to body fat percentage, they do have a rough correlation to the risk of disease that certain body fat percentages can pose.

B) Incorrect. The procedures for performing and analyzing skinfold measurements are quite rigorous, and the data can be correlated with the percentage of an individual's body fat.

C) Incorrect. As with answer choice B, the data gathered through these measurements can be correlated with the percentage of an individual's body fat.

D) Incorrect. Both of these techniques are fairly complex; they also correlate with body fat percentage.

97. **A)** Incorrect. The *S* in the SMART acronym does not stand for *start*.

B) Incorrect. The *S* in the SMART acronym does not stand for *strong*.

C) **Correct.** The *S* in the SMART acronym stands for *specific*.

D) Incorrect. The *S* in the SMART acronym does not stand for *silly*.

98. **A)** Incorrect. The 5-10-5 test is used to assess lateral speed and agility.

B) **Correct.** The 5-10-5 shuttle test is used to assess 180-degree-direction change ability, horizontal speed, and agility.

C) Incorrect. The LEFT is used to assess an individual's ability to run in the sagittal and frontal plane.

D) Incorrect. The long jump test is used to assess maximal horizontal jumping.

99. **A)** Incorrect. Quadriceps flexibility is not assessed during the sit-and-reach test.

B) Incorrect. Shoulder flexibility is not assessed during the sit-and-reach test.

C) **Correct.** The sit-and-reach test assesses lower back and hamstring flexibility.

D) The sit-and-reach test is a flexibility assessment, not a strength assessment.

100. **A)** Incorrect. Balance is controlled instability.

B) Incorrect. Sprinting is forward movement.

C) **Correct.** Plyometrics promotes force production with explosive upward or forward movement.

D) Incorrect. Sliding is a movement pattern utilized in advanced core training.

101. **A)** Incorrect. This is a benefit of stretching.

B) Incorrect. This is a benefit of proper nutrition.

C) **Correct.** Building lean mass through resistance training allows for more caloric expenditure as muscles burn more calories than fat.

D) Incorrect. Speed, agility, and quickness training attribute to a longer stride.

102. **A)** Incorrect. Hydraulic machines use compressed air or water to create resistance.

B) Incorrect. Cardio machines use incline or electronic resistance.

C) **Correct.** Cam machines use weight, pulley friction, and gravity to create resistance.

D) Incorrect. These machines use air only to create resistance.

103. A) Incorrect. This is not the definition of a training plateau.

B) Incorrect. A training plateau does not refer to the described training design.

C) Correct. A training plateau occurs when the client is not seeing any benefits from the exercise program due to lack of overload.

D) Incorrect. This describes the principle of progression.

104. **A) Correct.** Joints can be described as the fulcrum of a lever system in the human body.

B) Incorrect. Bones are better described as the lever arms in a lever system.

C) Incorrect. Muscles are better described as the muscular force used to lift the resistance.

D) Incorrect. Organs are a structure of the biological hierarchy of the human body.

105. **A) Correct.** Scheduling negativity is a tool that facilitates belief in oneself and combats self-doubt.

B) Incorrect. Positivity is the opposite of the scheduling negativity tool.

C) Incorrect. Goal-setting is a tool to help a person keep focused on his or her goals.

D) Incorrect. Exercise goals help a person keep focused on his or her goals.

106. A) Incorrect. This is a third-class lever.

B) Incorrect. This is a third-class lever.

C) Correct. This is one of the only first-class levers on the body where the skull meets the C1 vertebrae.

D) Incorrect. This is one of the only examples of a second-class lever of the body.

107. **A) Correct.** These exercises focus in prime mover force production.

B) Incorrect. These moves do not focus on building muscle or tendon strength.

C) Incorrect. These moves do not focus on building correct form or reducing body fat.

D) Incorrect. These are types of exercises not a training continuum.

108. A) Incorrect. The client may still be learning how to master the techniques of the exercises in the program and could overtrain by progressing further.

B) Incorrect. The cognitive phase shows that the client is still struggling to complete the task and requires further practice to eliminate compensatory movements.

C) Incorrect. If the client is still having significant delayed-onset muscle soreness, the client is still achieving overload and should not progress yet.

D) Correct. The client has mastered or nearly mastered the training technique and is ready to increase the difficulty of the workout through the manipulation of training variables.

109. A) Incorrect. Liability cannot be prevented entirely by paperwork, and the medical history form is not an exception.

B) Correct. The medical history form helps the trainer decide whether the client requires a physician's clearance in order to begin exercising.

C) Incorrect. The client's interest in exercising cannot be determined by the medical history form.

D) Incorrect. Determining workout intensity is not the purpose of the medical history form.

110. A) Incorrect. This is an insufficient calorie reduction to lose one pound of fat per week. The addition of exercise would help to spur significant weight loss.

B) Incorrect. Many individuals would not be able to sustain this frequency of activity, and this may not create enough of a caloric deficit for significant weight loss.

C)   Incorrect. This would be difficult to sustain and could cause nutrient deficiencies.

D)   Correct. These are sustainable changes in behavior that would create a calorie deficit of around 4,000 kcal/week—enough to lose a little over one pound per week.

111. A)   Incorrect. The two components impact one another.

B)   Incorrect. Force decreases as time increases.

C)   Incorrect. There is a change to force with a concurrent change in time.

D)   Correct. The force-time curve indicates that applied force decreases over time.

112. A)   Incorrect. Power is the application of force × velocity, where velocity is necessary.

B)   Incorrect. Force is mass × acceleration.

C)   Correct. This is the definition of strength.

D)   Incorrect. Endurance refers to the ability of the muscle to apply force for multiple efforts.

113. A)   Incorrect. Reassessing clients will help keep them committed to their goals.

B)   Incorrect. Reassessing client goals is a great time to reevaluate goals that were selected at the initial assessment.

C)   Incorrect. The reassessment period serves as an opportunity to modify the exercise program.

D)   Correct. When reassessing clients, it is important to keep the same test protocol.

114. **A)   Correct.** Fast feet and A-skips are ideal dynamic warm-ups because they focus on increasing the range of motion for the lower body while adding quickness and footwork.

B)   Incorrect. Fast feet and A-skips are not ideal for cooldowns as they are high intensity.

C)   Incorrect. Fast feet and A-skips are to be done in shorter bursts. Endurance focuses on longer cardio bouts of training.

D)   Incorrect. Fast feet and A-skips do not represent static stretching protocols.

115. A)   Incorrect. It is less intense than anaerobic endurance training.

B)   Incorrect. It is typically longer duration, and beginner programs should start at twenty to thirty minutes.

C)   Incorrect. Steady state is not specific and can cause increased influence of the wrong type of muscle fibers for power athletes.

D)   Correct. Steady-state activity is an appropriate form of cardiovascular activity for long-distance runners such as cross-country runners.

116. A)   Incorrect. Oxygen is used to form ATP in the aerobic energy system.

B)   Correct. Creatine phosphate is used to create ATP molecules in the anaerobic energy system.

C)   Incorrect. Lactic acid is a byproduct of anaerobic exercise.

D)   Incorrect. Acetyl CoA forms ATP in the presence of oxygen in the Krebs cycle.

117. A)   Incorrect. This individual has three cardiovascular risk factors.

B)   Incorrect. A low-risk assessment is not correct, given the multiple cardiovascular risk factors.

C)   Incorrect. An intermediate-risk assessment is too low for this client.

D)   Correct. This individual would be considered high risk and would require a physician's clearance to begin an exercise program.

118. A)   Incorrect. While the push jerk is considered a more advanced move, it is not the direct progression.

B)   Incorrect. The upright row targets the shoulders and trapezius, not the lower body.

C)   **Correct.** The still-leg deadlift is the next progression, as the user would use the full range of motion allowing the barbell to go all the way to the floor, as opposed to stopping mid-shin.

D)   Incorrect. The inverted hamstring would be a rather dynamic stretch for the Romanian deadlift.

119. A)   **Correct.** The metronome should be set to ninety-six beats per minute.

B)   Incorrect. One hundred and eight beats per minute is not proper test procedure.

C)   Incorrect. There are twenty-four steps performed per minute, but the metronome is set to ninety-six beats per minute.

D)   Incorrect. Forty-eight beats per minute is not proper test procedure.

120. A)   Incorrect. The 1.5-mile run measures aerobic power.

B)   **Correct.** The three-hundred yard shuttle test measures anaerobic capacity.

C)   Incorrect. The Rockport walk test is used to estimate aerobic capacity, or VO2 max.

D)   Incorrect. The twelve-minute run test is used to determine an individual's ability to use oxygen pathways for energy while running.

121. A)   Incorrect. This is referring to catabolism.

B)   Incorrect. This is the body's energy source, ATP.

C)   **Correct.** Anabolism is a metabolic process in which molecules are built up.

D)   Incorrect. This is referring to oxygen uptake.

122. A)   Incorrect. Weights should be kept light for children so they can work on technique.

B)   Incorrect. While strength is not the primary focus, it is one of the benefits of training children.

C)   **Correct.** Improving technique and emphasizing form is most important when training children.

D)   Incorrect. Power is an advanced benefit of exercise and should not be the primary emphasis of a child's training routine.

123. A)   Incorrect. This is a compressed air or water resisted machine.

B)   Incorrect. This is an air propelled machine.

C)   Incorrect. This is a body weight exercise

D)   **Correct.** Dumbbells are considered free weights.

124. A)   Incorrect. Mentorships and observations are correct, but ownerships is not.

B)   **Correct.** Observations, internships, and mentorships are the three ways a new trainer can gain hands-on experience while on the job.

C)   Incorrect. Internships provide opportunities to gain knowledge and experience, but the other two methods, leaderships and ownerships, are not.

D)   Incorrect. Mentorships and internships are correct, but leaderships is not.

125. A)   Incorrect. Speed training is not the primary focus of cone drills. Resisted and assisted sprints focus on speed.

B)   **Correct.** Cone drills focus on reaction time and direction change.

C)   Incorrect. Agility training is not the primary focus of cone drills. Ladders drills focus on agility.

D)   Incorrect. Resistance training is not the primary focus of cone drills. Weight machines and free weights focus on resistance training.

126. A)   Incorrect. It helps to develop type II muscle fibers.

B)   Incorrect. It is already a tough workout and will cause further soreness.

C) **Correct.** This intensity level is good for improving lactate threshold and movement speed.

D) Incorrect. Steady state, long-distance cardiovascular activity helps to lower resting heart rate.

127. A) Correct. Athletes tend to have more strength and coordination when starting a fitness program.

B) Incorrect. Athletes tend to have more strength when starting a fitness program.

C) Incorrect. Athletes tend to have more coordination when starting a fitness program.

D) Incorrect. Untrained individuals tend to fatigue faster.

128. A) Incorrect. The carotid artery is not the preferred landmark for determining resting heart rate.

B) Incorrect. The femoral artery is not the preferred landmark for determining resting heart rate.

C) Incorrect. The brachial artery is not the preferred landmark for determining resting heart rate.

D) Correct. The radial pulse is the preferred landmark for determining resting heart rate due to the safety of its location and ease of finding it.

129. A) Correct. The systolic number represents the pressure in the arterial system after the heart contracts.

B) Incorrect. The point at which the pulse can no longer be felt occurs when the cuff is inflated 20 – 30 mmHg past the pulse point.

C) Incorrect. The fading away of the pulse represents the diastolic pressure reading.

D) Incorrect. The sphygmomanometer is the device used to determine blood pressure.

130. A) Incorrect. Training frequency can remain the same during pregnancy as long as the mother is healthy and cleared for exercise.

B) Incorrect. Resistance training is still beneficial for expectant mothers.

C) Correct. Rest periods between sets should be increased to prevent overheating or excessive intensity.

D) Incorrect. Modifications should be made for abdominal exercises, but they should not be completely eliminated from the exercise program.

131. A) Incorrect. The lifter should only use a spotter if their form is correct and they should be doing most of the work.

B) Correct. The lifter should be able to maintain core integrity and good form at all times.

C) Incorrect. Like answer choice A, the lifter should always have correct form first and foremost.

D) Incorrect. If a lifter doesn't feel secure with the weight lifted, they should not go up in weight.

132. A) Incorrect. Human growth hormone is a peptide hormone.

B) Correct. Testosterone is a steroid hormone.

C) Incorrect. Human chorionic gonadotropin is a peptide hormone.

D) Incorrect. Luteinizing hormone is a peptide hormone.

133. A) Incorrect. Nutrition is not an aspect of the triad.

B) Incorrect. Exercise is not an aspect of the triad.

C) Incorrect. None of these three are correct.

D) Correct. The female athlete triad consists of amenorrhea, disordered eating, and osteoporosis.

134. A) Incorrect. Clients should complete the PAR-Q.

B) Incorrect. The medical disclosure is one form that clients should be sure to complete.

C) Correct. The demographic form is not required for clients.

D) Incorrect. The client must complete the contract.

135. A) Incorrect. Level of soreness is not a proper differentiation between DOMS and overtraining symptoms; both can elicit the same degree of soreness.

B) Incorrect. Overtraining and DOMS can occur in the same muscles.

C) Incorrect. DOMS is a normal physiological response to overloading the muscles, whereas overtraining is an abnormal response due to inadequate rest.

D) **Correct.** DOMS typically involves acute soreness, whereas overtraining involves chronic soreness.

136. A) Incorrect. Some poorly controlled studies have reported positive results. However, rigorous studies have found that Garcinia cambogia does not cause weight loss.

B) Incorrect. This can lead to overheating, dehydration, and dangerous stress to the heart. Any weight loss experienced is also mostly water.

C) Incorrect. This method does not provide adequate carbohydrates to fuel exercise and can strain the kidneys due to excess nitrogen excretion, resulting in buildup of toxic keto acids in the blood because of the incomplete metabolism of fat.

D) **Correct.** This method uses moderate behavioral changes that are sustainable for a lifetime, which is the key to losing weight and keeping it off.

137. A) Incorrect. The hip adductor complex is part of the core, as it supports trunk rotation and posture.

B) Incorrect. The erector spinae is part of the core, as it supports trunk rotation and posture.

C) **Correct.** The biceps brachii are the muscles located in the anterior side of the arms.

D) Incorrect. The internal obliques are part of the core, supporting trunk rotation and posture.

138. A) Incorrect. The cardiovascular system changes with age.

B) Incorrect. Maximal heart rate does not increase with age.

C) **Correct.** Maximal heart rate decreases with age.

D) Incorrect. The risk of atherosclerosis increases with age.

139. A) **Correct.** Skinfold measurements are the most commonly used form of body fat testing due to the ease, convenience, and low cost of performing this method of assessment.

B) Incorrect. Body mass index does not determine body fat; it only determines what an individual's weight should be in proportion to height.

C) Incorrect. Air displacement plethysmography is highly accurate, but it is not the most commonly used method.

D) Incorrect. Circumference measurements determine the girth of body segments but not the body fat percentage.

140. A) **Correct.** A shorter duration may be necessary to build up cardiovascular capacity before advancing to longer sessions.

B) Incorrect. Though these are the general guidelines for individuals starting a cardiovascular exercise routine, it will likely be too advanced for someone with COPD.

C) Incorrect. This recommendation is for intermediate to advanced exercisers with no current medical concerns.

D) Incorrect. COPD patients benefit greatly from cardiovascular training and should not completely eliminate it.

141. A) Incorrect. A feeling of pressure to maintain a lean body weight is a feature of anorexia.

B) **Correct.** Anorexia causes an aversion to eating, not an insatiable desire for food.

C) Incorrect. Inadequate dietary intake causes nutrient deficiencies.

D) Incorrect. Anorexic individuals drastically limit caloric intake.

142. A) Incorrect. Unless the trainer is working as a mobile fitness trainer, gyms should have plenty of equipment.

B) Correct. Gyms do not have personal liability coverage for personal trainers.

C) Incorrect. While it is important to have a computer, if employed at a gym, a trainer can manage without one.

D) Incorrect. While these are always good to have handy, trainers at gyms tend to get plenty of leads without business cards; some gyms may also provide business cards for their trainers.

143. A) Incorrect. High intensity aerobic training will not necessarily decrease the risk of a fall.

B) Incorrect. Swimming requires little balance but is a great low impact joint exercise.

C) Incorrect. Improved maximal upper body strength will not necessarily decrease the risk of a fall.

D) Correct. Exercises to improve balance during activities of daily living, such as box step-ups, will help to reduce the risk of a fall in older adults.

144. A) Incorrect. Anorexia nervosa is characterized by an unwillingness to eat enough.

B) Incorrect. Obesity is extreme excess weight and does not necessarily entail any compensatory behavior.

C) Correct. Bulimia nervosa involves binge eating with extreme compensatory behavior.

D) Incorrect. The female athlete triad consists of anorexia nervosa, amenorrhea, and osteoporosis.

145. **A) Correct.** Physiological assessments should be performed in a resting state before a flexibility assessment takes place.

B) Incorrect. Aerobic assessments should be performed after a flexibility assessment.

C) Incorrect. Muscular endurance assessments should be performed after physiological assessments have been completed.

D) Incorrect. Strength assessments should be performed after physiological assessments have been completed.

146. A) Incorrect. A recent history of myocardial infarction is an example of an absolute contraindication.

B) Incorrect. Suffering from unstable angina is an example of an absolute contraindication in a client.

C) Incorrect. When a patient exhibits uncontrolled symptomatic heart failure, it is an example of an absolute contraindication.

D) Correct. Severe high blood pressure is a relative contraindication.

147. A) Incorrect. Muscle imbalance is inconsistency in a muscle's length around a joint.

B) Incorrect. The term *proprietary* relates to the ownership of something.

C) Incorrect. Core control relates to an individual's ability to control the muscles of the core during an exercise.

D) Correct. Proprioception describes having a sense of the body and its relationship to the surrounding space; it also refers to the ability to balance.

148. A) Incorrect. Working the muscles, even at a lighter load, can continue to cause overtraining symptoms.

B) Incorrect. Symptoms of overtraining can still be caused by working the muscles at a lighter volume.

C) Correct. Temporary cessation of exercise and resting before restarting exercise helps the client overcome overtraining symptoms.

D) Incorrect. Cardiovascular exercise can still result in overtraining symptoms.

149. A) Incorrect. All trainers should stay up-to-date on fitness research.

B)   Incorrect. All certified personal trainers must be in good standing with a certifying agency.

C)   **Correct.** Punctuality is a professional standard that trainers should follow, but it is not a requirement for trainer certification.

D)   Incorrect. Holding a valid CPR/AED certification is a requirement for all certified professional trainers.

150. A)   Incorrect. DOMS stands for *Delayed Onset Muscle Soreness.*

B)   **Correct.** FAST stands for *Face, Arms, Speech, and Time*; reviewing these features helps to determine if someone is having a stroke.

C)   Incorrect. EPOC stands for *Excess Post-exercise Oxygen Consumption.*

D)   Incorrect. RICE stands for *Rest, Ice, Compression, Elevation.*

Made in the USA
Lexington, KY
02 June 2017